Too many truths are hidden.

PRODUCTS
OF
OUR
ENVIRONMENT

Too many lies are taught.

by Ray Stone

PRODUCTS OF OUR ENVIRONMENT

© 2013 Ra One Publications LLC

E-mail: ra1publications@gmail.com
Web: www.raonebooks.com
Phone: (313) 559-6200

- *Speaking Engagements*
- *Special Order Needs*
- *Life Coaching Packages*
- *General Inquiries*

Cover Design & Layout: **Ray Stone & Michael Angelo Chester**
Editor: **Ann Houston**
Photo Credits: **Rashid Bey**
Rear Cover Photo: **Selfie**

Manufactured in the US Republic (Northwest Amexem)
10 9 8 7 6 5 4 3 2 1
For Library of Congress Data, See Publisher

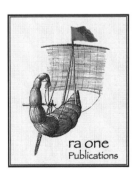

Dedicated to my ancestors:

My father **Benjamin Stone,** my uncles **Arthur Beard** (*Uncle Magic*) and **Charles Raymond Beard**—my aunts **Phyllis Hall** (*Nana*), **Barbara Nelthrope** and **Wanda Beard**—and my awesome grandmother **Emma Beard** (*'Big Gran'*).

Rest in power **Alan Sharpe, Laura Bailey, Mrs. Lonzena Felix, Van Wiley Sr.**

Gone way too soon **Desma Johnson.**

You are all missed.

WELCOME TO PRODUCTS OF OUR ENVIRONMENT
There are a number of useful topics for you to explore!

WELCOME TO PRODUCTS OF OUR ENVIRONMENT
There are a number of useful topics for you to explore!

Section 5: Change

Section 6: Nurturing/Balance/Judgment

Section 7: Spirituality/Meditation

Section 8: Business/Goals/Deep Insight

Products of Our Environment

MESSAGE TO THE READER

Peace and love,

Please understand that the information in this book is not intended to be prescriptive in nature. The author/publisher can assume absolutely no responsibility for the improper application or interpretation of the ideas outlined in this book. Understand that all actions pursued as a result of this material are at the sole risk of the reader. The author/publisher is not qualified to offer anything other than a humble opinion and some advice. Life is about us all finding our own balance. Although we are all connected, we are on unique journeys as well. You are encouraged to do your own research and explore some of the recommended material. This book is offering you some less expensive, considerably safer and more natural options to consider.

This material is not in any way meant to bring slander to any particular product, corporation or government agency. (However, in the name of free speech, I do want to say f*ck Monsanto!) It is only my strong suggestion that we at least take time to read and closely evaluate the information provided right on the bottles of anything that we use in our homes. We should expect and demand nothing less than the highest standard of quality. Our families deserve that.

One of the ultimate aims of P.O.E. is to help re-instill the value of production into every individual, home and community in America. We need to learn to make things and begin to trust in each other more and depend less on corporations.

The author is merely a playing the role of messenger. This material points out some practical things that we all could stand to reevaluate and investigate in some capacity. The hope is that it will help invite some new ideas and new energy into your homes and lives.

This unique little D-I-Y/Variety book from Ra One Publications should do nothing less than provide some nourishing food for thought. Thank you for your support!

(If you need to add salt to that food for thought it would do you well to not use the **man made** regular table salt. Use real sea salt instead. Commercial white salt is actually a waste product of the petroleum industry that is bleached and full of chemicals. That stuff has no place in the body Temple. That is why they say salt is bad for you and causes the high blood pressure. *No bueno!* Sea salt however is a **product of nature** that naturally contains trace minerals and it can be useful in a number of different ways. Replace white table salt with Celtic sea salt or even better a rich colorful sea salt, like Hawaiian or Himalayan. This book is about little stuff like that and ***mucho mas!***)

Products of Our Environment

THIS IS THE TIME FOR CHANGE

Peace and love! Welcome to Products of Our Environment.

POE asks readers to re-evaluate some of the products we use daily on our bodies and in our households. We will examine some practical ways to cut some corners in that area in order to save money and reduce the overall amount of chemicals we are exposed to at home.

It is an unfortunate fact that we all live within the confines of this capitalistic, corporate dominated society. What we have to make sure that the corporations do not live inside of us and run our households. We have gotten so far away from the old fashioned ways of our grand and great grandparents. Most of our elders had an idea of how to grow their own food and had an arsenal of tools to fix and make things last forever, handing them down to us. This generation the M.O. is to go out and buy cheap Chinese made crap from 24-hour mega stores that sell everything – including food.

Overall, we have become too dependent on the system.

We eat far more processed, machine food than we do hand made food. It's not even close anymore. I saw a timeline post of children in Asia ordering and eating food from a popular fast food chain out of a vending machine. That is a fitting image because that is how far the corporations want to take us away from humanity. They are getting there too. Look at where we are today. **Everyday we use products (and eat "foods") full of artificial colors, flavors and fragrances.** We're really comfortable with cheap, artificial things. At this rate that is all the future generations will ever know about. They will grow up thinking that we are supposed to get everything that we need to sustain ourselves from the local superstore.

Who is going to teach the young girls to knit blankets, bake cakes or make biscuits from scratch? Where will we find a new generation of bakers, farmers, gardeners and seamstresses? At the rate we're going things like that will soon become lost arts. Unfortunately there is no smartphone app for that.

We have generally become too dependent on products. We exist in such an artificial world that we are losing touch with nature. We are losing our natural human instincts and relationship with the land. How well could we even manage our home if suddenly there were no superstores in strip malls in every community? Would we still be able to clean, wash, eat and live normally? Are our lives oversaturated by the same commercial name brands? Take a look through your cabinets, then look at the picture on page 42 and re-evaluate that.

Please keep in mind that this material is created only to enlighten and give us all some things to think about. It is not about looking down upon or judging anyone.

There is a thin line that we all must walk. I'm no better than anyone else. I am even typing this on my mandatory MacBook and I'm that hippie that wants to be free, sovereign and off the grid – but definitely *with* the latest iPhone and my power toothbrush for sure, lol! So I know what it's like out here. The commerce game is real. I am in a personal battle with the corporate system too. We all are. **POE** is here to provide some easy, safe and affordable ammunition.

As anyone who read my first book knows, one thing I have been diligent about is keeping corporate food out of my being. I have taken myself completely out of the fast food, commercial food and chain restaurant loop. I strongly encourage everyone to work towards doing the same. Overall I try to do as little business with chain restaurants and any large commercial retailers as possible. It has become one of my personal goals to not rely on the megastores and common drug store chains. I try to totally ignore them and not even step foot inside them. I have found a great form of freedom in taking that step alone.

It's time that we all take the next step in our lifestyle transition. We all need to give some thought to the products that we commonly use in and on our bodies and inside our homes. **Most of us loyally use and trust the same brands of cosmetics that we grew up using** or go with the leading brands, assuming that they are safe to use. One would think that is a safe assumption, but in America it is not. As you read on you will find that we are putting a great deal of trust in a handful of huge corporations who are abusing it.

When we do all of our shopping at commercial stores then it is very likely that the same few corporations are dominating so much of our lives. At damn near every house in the neighborhood everyone has the same brands of dressings and condiments. In the fridge we have: a Ranch dressing, a light Raspberry Vinaigrette, Thousand Island dressing, some Jello and cheese slices. The cabinets are stocked with peanut butter, crackers, cookies and mac &

cheese and **all** of it is from the ***same*** damn company! That is giving them far too much access to your home and your body temple. That corporation is basically sustaining you completely. That is too much.

Just like we all need human contact and interaction – understand that **we also need a level of humanity involved in the way we care for ourselves too.** It is important that we support local producers of hand made things. The value of humanity is priceless.

POE will show us how to easily find and make some safe and effective alternatives. Lets discuss taking a different approach towards commercial products going forward. Now is the time to come out of your comfort zone and make a few changes in your daily routine. Of course we all love the convenience, prices and accessibility of the sell everything superstore – but I urge you to begin to depend on those types of places less. They are supplying us with too much.

Commercial products are all mass-produced. Machine made. Nothing created like that has any human or nature elements involved with it – therefore there cannot be any uplifting energy in those products. They are cold with no soul inside them. They are filled with corporate energy and that is not an energy that we want to be filling our homes (or bodies & minds) with.

Just like they say the contents of your fridge can say a lot about your health – the soaps, cleansers, fresheners and detergents used in our homes can speak volumes as well. In fact processed foods and commercial cleansers even share some of the same ingredients these days.

It is common for us to store very strong chemical cleansers at home – like chlorine bleach for instance. But why do we need all of that – why should such a vast arsenal of (toxic) cleansers reside under the sinks? **Have we become too comfortable and frivolous using products that contain toxic ingredients inside our homes?** We don't seem to mind using them – often without proper ventilation – around our children, pets and plants without thinking twice about it.

Consider the fact that everything we put down our drains will eventually become a part of the municipal water supply. Using more earth friendly products is not only better for us individually – it's better for us all.

We should assume the responsibility of making our own products. Every trip to the superstore supports corporations that are well known for bad things – like animal testing, chemical dumping and worker/land exploitation. Our dollars support the same corporations that are working to monopolize the food industry and keep us in the dark in this country. Look how much money they spent to keep California's Prop 37, which would require manufacturers to label foods with GMO ingredients, from passing. These are not the entities that we want to give our support to any longer. And we don't have to!

That is why some education and change in our daily operation and perspective is necessary. This book will point us in the direction of some natural products of our environment that we can easily utilize and take advantage of. Take heed. Knowledge is power.

Now, let's get to it…

WELCOME TO THE ARTIFICIAL WORLD

I had a chance to sit and talk at length with my big brother Mike at our annual family Retreat a few years back. It's held at a small campground in western Michigan. I appreciated the chance to kick it with him, especially at a late hour on a silent night. That is my prime time.

The serene quiet of the campground and the energy from the moonlit sky flooded with stars – which of course are not visible in the smoggy city – provided a great natural backdrop for conversation. In what has become the normal routine of life, I rarely get the opportunity to talk with my brother or most of my other extended family members on that level, especially at that hour. The pace of the artificial world is just too fast! We catch up with each other on the so-called holidays and at the other scheduled family functions, but those times are usually just long enough to discuss the local sports teams or the most recent big story on the news – the same stuff that everyone is talking about. There is always something remarkable going on in the Detroit headlines.

Some isolated time away from news, televisions and the stresses of the busy city, surrounded by the noise of busy crickets instead of traffic, provides a chance to share deeper thoughts. I was local beer amped up and told him all about this book. Focusing particularly on the real world versus the artificial one.

I broke it down for a good hour or so, going in about the whole idea of the artificial world, (it was slated to be a whole book at that time). I patiently waited for his reaction to all of that. I know it's a lot to take in. He smiled really big and laughed out loud. He was quietly pondering for what seemed like a long moment before saying anything at all. I'm sure he was exhausted too.

As the sounds of nature grew louder, he was still visibly in chess player like thought. We stood to walk towards the cabins and he smiled again. Finally he simply said, "I like it".

After one more pause for a big, spontaneous yawn he added, "You know…it kinda sounds like that movie."

I quickly nodded and gave him a hard pound. I immediately knew just what movie he meant – and I knew he had felt me. That was quite a few years ago. I can't wait to finally hand him a copy of P.O.E. I was very thankful for that time and space to share that kind of real dialogue with him.

"Yes," I enthusiastically confirmed. Way too turned up for that hour.

"It *is*!"

America is the Matrix!

The way that corporate dollars and commercial marketing affect how we live today is completely unreal. One of the most glaring examples of the Artificial World is in the hospitals and our babies.

What exactly is the priority of our hospitals? It seems that it is to create and produce more patients. It's an ugly and deadly business. Why the hell are fast food restaurants allowed INSIDE or anywhere near hospitals? There should be a safe zone. Speaking of food, why would they not serve decent meals to patients at the hospitals – like soups and herbal teas? Doesn't that make perfect sense? Why are there flocks of eager pharmaceutical sales reps wooing doctors into over prescribing every new and largely untested chemical drug?

This can't be real. People would never go for that, we are smarter than that. Aren't we?

For instance, it just baffles me that a bright pink baby lotion can proudly boast being the '#1 choice of hospitals'!

I was completely shocked when I turned the bottle over to read the ingredients:

PROPYLENE GLYCOL, MYRISTYL MYRISTATE, GLYCERYL STEARATE, OLEIC ACID, STEARIC ACID, POLYSORBATE 61, C12-15 ALKYL BENZOATE, DIMETHICONE, ISOPROPYL PALMITATE, SORBITAN STEARATE, CETYL ALCOHOL, SYNTHETIC BEESWAX, STEARYL ALCOHOL, BENZYL ALCOHOL, CARBOMER, FRAGRANCE, METHYLPAROBEN, PROPYLPARABEN, BUTYLPARABEN, BHT, SODIUM HYDROXIDE, RED 33.

Wait a minute…that is what the **hospital** recommends for fucking *babies*? A bunch of crazy looking chemicals?! Huh?

If a scientist in a lab coat came up to a mother with some of those chemicals in a test tube and tried to rub it on her child's skin, she would rightfully fight them to the death. But if it's all mixed in a pretty bottle in the isle of the store she will pay money for it and rub it all over her child who she loves more than anything in the world. It is deceitful and sickening, at best.

That, (and other unnatural substances like the sucrose in the water that they give newborns in the hospitals), become the initiation and inception of the artificial person.

A little baby is for all practical purposes, perfect. And so very delicate! Just the thought of taking that mixture of chemicals and smearing it on human skin is so unnatural! Look at that list of ingredients again slowly! Does that look like something made for human skin – much less a baby's skin? Hell no!

We are nature's creations. It only makes sense that we maintain ourselves with natural things! Everything that we need is already here and provided by our Creator. It all exists in nature.

In our product driven society, we introduce our systems to artificial tastes and chemicals that are not natural to this planet. Surely there were no such bright colorful foods and products 500 or 1000 years ago – and babies have been turning out just fine without it.

Gradually, these products have replaced nature in the daily routine of our lives. We have used many of these brands our entire lives. We love the smell and associate it with good memories. But we have to remember that these man made products created in laboratories are merely poor imitations of natural things. The smell is totally artificial! It's not real.

Man-made imitations are no comparison to God's creations. We have to be more conscious of what we put on and in our bodies.

The skin in fact is our body's largest organ. The pores of our skin are actually 4 times more absorbent than the mouth. Meaning something rubbed on our skin reaches the bloodstream 4 times faster than if we had eaten it. Therefore anything we put on our skin we should be able to eat it! Could you imagine putting all of those chemicals into a baby's bloodstream all at once? Damn! It's crazy. **It simply has to change. We have to be more aware and in control of what goes in and on our body temples. We should not even expect to be healthy with all that unknown stuff entering our bloodstreams at one time.**

I am not a biochemist or an expert, but I am smart enough to know that chemicals like that are not natural or welcome in the human system. It is safe to assume that eventually using too many artificial chemical ingredients could lead to health complications down the line. The body is not equipped to deal with this artificial madness.

> *"They do not come from the ground where (things) grow – those things come from a laboratory. If you keep (using) laboratory creations, as opposed to nature's gifts, you will surely end up needing laboratory drugs and medicines."*
>
> —E.L.Y.G.A.D.

Nothing new that has been created in a laboratory is any better than nature. Get out of that store! Use natural substances that are the same today as they were 200 years ago. There was no cancer epedemic 200 years ago. There were no neon pink or electric blue lotions and soaps either. Maybe that is no coincidence. Why even continue to take that kind of risk?

This is the time that we should return to the old fashioned ways and stick with natural things like: Shea Butter, Coconut Oil, Aloe Vera gel, Almond Oil, Black Seed Oil, Oz Oil, etc. – those are substances that can enter your bloodstream more seamlessly, creating less confusion in your system. If you can't eat it, you should not put it on your skin.

The more natural and less artificial things we use, the better it is for our health, immune systems. It is better for the earth itself. Natural products enhance and highlight our inner beauty and subtly remind us of our origin in nature.

Artificial ingredients simply cause confusion in the system. It is that confusion which sets the table for dis-ease in the body.

There are artificial colors and flavors in MOST commercial products, especially the ones marketed to children. Read the ingredients of everything before you feed it to your children. Artificial colors like **Red #40, Yellow #6** or **Blue #1** – are widely BANNED from use (without big warning labels) in European countries due to their health risks. Yet in the U.S., they remain literally a daily occurrence in our children's diet.

It is up to us to protect our households. The corporations here just want us to set that table for disease very early on in our lives – so the greedy American system can slowly eat us alive.

LITTLE BABY BLUE SUEDE SHOES

The human body goes through a drastic change from the naturally protective barrier of the mother's womb, quickly into this artificial world of chemical drugs.

Very early on we start layering our bodies with unnatural chemicals. Compare that to the coating someone would put on a pair of brand new suede shoes. They use a chemical mixture to protect the suede from the rain and other natural elements.

The symbol of that lotion serves as an initiation, exposing our delicate bodies early on to the world of chemical ingredients that will be ubiquitous throughout our lifetimes. Welcome to the artificial world!

Early on the introduction of many crazy ass ingredients like **BHT (Butylated hydroxytoluene)** which is a preservative in food and also used in cosmetics, pharmaceuticals, jet fuels, rubber, petroleum products, electrical transformer oil and of course embalming fluid! That is totally ridiculous!

It is only in this corrupt capitalistic society that something like that would be an ingredient in any product recommended for our children! Hospital recommended at that! This just can't be real. But it is.

We all know that the #1 choice of hospitals is there for only one reason. The company has invested millions of dollars to have that printed on their bottles – not because it is the safest and best quality product available. What kind of society do we live in where everything – even our hospitals and the trust of the people – can be bought?

That is an example of how the commerce game assuming control of us. It is not so ironic that the commercial products like that lotion and what they stand for actually embody the term c.r.e.a.m.

> *"Cash Rules Everything Around Me... Cream! Get the money, dollar dollar bill y'all."*
> —Wu Tang

The hospitals cannot encourage or promote natural things! That is not how the system works. They are highly trained to steer us – the cattle – in the direction of profit producing PRODUCTS.

They would never suggest that we heat some distilled water with some raw Shea or cocoa butter, add some vitamin E, coconut milk/oil or aloe vera juice to create your own safe moisturizing lotions at home. They don't want us to think like that, so they train the doctors not to think like that. We seem to think that doctor is God. They have trained us too. Ultimately, over the years we have all been led very far away from nature and natural thoughts.

There is no money to be made in promoting nature or natural body care. So instead they will have us use crazy chemicals on our children and then when they come up with a skin rash (surprise, surprise) – they will happily prescribe some other chemical concoction to treat that. Take this prescription to the pharmacy. That's the cycle. It goes on for a lifetime. It has become the American way.

Today the dis-eases get more serious because the products have become even more artificial.

What we have to do to counteract that is at least try not to depend on commercial manufacturers. Get into the practice of going to the superstore as little as possible. Cut down on trips to the huge local supermarket and the corner pharmacy. Try to limit the things you need from those places. Stick with a smaller circle of farmers markets, co-ops and local venues.

The overall focus of the health system is not health and nutrition. **The whole system, if not our whole society, has become completely product driven.** Today the pharmaceutical business is very, very lucrative. Pharmacies have never experienced a recession, they continue to spring up everywhere. All kinds of new pills pop up on the market for nearly every kind of symptom. These are experimental things with no long-term research done and a huge list of 'side' effects.

Corporations pay a lot of money to be considered "the leading brand" – because they know they can buy our trust. We think they would never recommend things that are unsafe for our delicate babies. Of course, who would want to harm a beautiful baby? But upon further review…maybe it is time we change that way of thinking. Let's take our trust away from corporations and learn to rely on nature and one other instead.

If we change our thought process, we can create a different reality. Remember that although pills and pharmacies do surround us – nature also surrounds us. There are many kinds of herbs and plants readily available to us for every symptom as well. We must learn to utilize those things and preserve and pass that knowledge to the future generations.

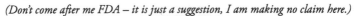

(Don't come after me FDA – it is just a suggestion, I am making no claim here.)

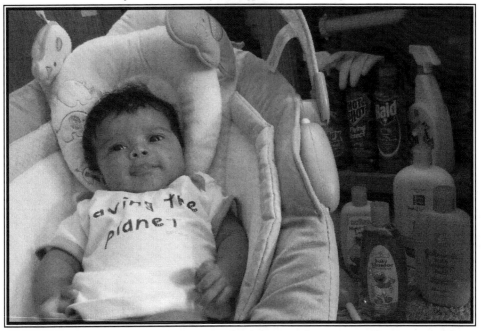

It is unfortunate that an arsenal commercial products with toxic ingredients surround our youth from day one. Our government allows and endorses it. In order to save our planet and ourselves, we should inch towards maintain our homes with more natural things going forward.

WE CAN LEARN A LOT BY LISTENING

Throughout my life, long talks with my mom have no doubt been the primary source of my education. Saturday mornings my Grandma would have them get up early to "general" clean up the house. She said for the windows that automatically meant: go fetch a pail of hot water, vinegar, a rag and some newspaper for the windows.

That is the only way they knew to clean windows.

Things certainly are different now aren't they? Today we are trained to look under the sink for the bottle of name brand "window cleaner" to spray on the glass. That is the instinct.

This is what I mean by us becoming products of our environment – we have been trained to think and operate just like the corporations would want us to. This has simply become a product driven society.

Today it feels so natural for us to use a named brand cleaner every time we need to clean the glass. We are off to the store to buy another bottle of it when we run out. But why continue to spend money on that if we actually don't need it? Especially when it is just an artificially colored, chemical mixture in a spray bottle? We could pour vinegar and water in our own spray bottle at a fraction of the cost – creating our own version. But…that leading brand is just become what we are used to today.

We have simply become too comfortable and careless with our use of toxic products.

Nobody pays much attention to the small print on the labels anymore. It warns us to keep out of the reach of children, but most of us keep it under the sink. It also explains that if ever it comes into contact with your eyes, or if it's swallowed – there can be serious danger. Call a physician or the Poison Control center type of danger. My question is: why we do we even need to deal with something poisonous just to clean up the house? It does not seem too wise.

Have you ever noticed how sometimes the smallest bit of mist from that spray ricochets gently into our faces as we fire away at the mirror in small non-ventilated bathrooms? It rains into our carpets and rugs and becomes a part of the home environment. Given what it is, that can't be too good!

All those warnings aren't printed on there for nothing. This is a pretty toxic and dangerous substance. We are just so accustomed to it that we don't look at it like that.

We will use it with our bare hands without even a second thought. We use it freely in the kitchen on the counters where our food touches. Spray it freely around our beloved babies, children and pets – it falls into the same carpets they'll crawl around on. We have simply become far too comfortable around these types of chemical based 'cleansers'.

If we think about it, vinegar and warm water is so much more eco friendly – and affordable. We could simply put that into our own spray bottle and use that. It is cheaper, safer, just as effective and just better all the way around. When we know we have better options available, we have to take it upon ourselves to start utilizing them and forming new habits going forward.

I know how it is though - it can be hard to break familiar habits. At everyone's crib in the hood growing up **PINE CLEANER** and **BLEACH** was the undisputed smell of "clean". I used to really love that pine smell.

At some point during my own personal naturalization, I just woke up and realized that is not actually pine scent at all. There is not a pine leaf or cone anywhere in sight or in the thought process when they make that cleanser. That is a complex mixture of chemical fragrances made to simulate the smell of fresh pine. It is totally artificially colored and scented.

Today that smell is so ridiculously strong to me and so blatantly chemically laced. I don't want to be in the same house with that crap anymore. Seriously.

But I can remember countless times dunking my bare hands into a hot bucket of warm pine soapy water to wring out my rag. We did the same thing with bleach water all the time. We even put a little bleach in the dishwater sometimes, as if that is necessary! What the hell? Are we talking about an Aids clinic or just our family's dirty dishes? The bleach smell would stay on our hands for hours and hours. That means it goes into the bloodstream. And that cannot be good! Don't let us bite our nails or rub our eyes after that you know? We are not giving these substances the proper respect.

Going forward, we need to be much more careful about dealing with chemically laced soaps and detergents. **Considering the amount of cancer and allergy/asthma type of symptoms today, cutting down the unnatural substances in the house is a really good idea any way you look at it.**

Stick with things that the body can recognize. Some simple combinations of vinegar, baking soda, lemon, food grade hydrogen peroxide, some essential oils and hot water can clean and disinfect our entire home quite easily. As I was talking to people about this book I realize that most people know that already, it came up in almost every conversation. Yet they still have a rainbow colored arsenal of products under the sink. I don't get it.

Using natural alternatives will not only save us money. More importantly, it saves our families from the constant exposure to harsh chemicals at home. Again if anyone living with us suffers from asthma/allergy/sinus type symptoms, it makes perfect sense to start removing some of the unnatural ingredients from the home environment. Make sure that your home is a safe and peaceful place.

This is an absolutely great time to return to some old fashioned ways of operating. We can use this time to teach the youth to regain the mentality of making food, cleansers and medicines inside the home.

We should begin transitioning our homes slowly and easily. Make a window cleaner when you run out of the spray next time. Make a cough syrup at home next time your child gets that little cough from the kids at school.

Start listening to elders and jot down their southern remedies. It is time to revert back to using things made with your human loving energy. We have to stop running to the local pharmacies and dollar stores daily for more and more toxic commercial products.

CHEMICALS IN COSMETICS

Ladies really set the tone of health in the household. In most homes, we rely on moms to do the bulk of the grocery shopping and cooking – plus take on the role of healers of the family. Those are all very important jobs.

We appreciate the things you do ladies, and we want the Queens of this earth to remain healthy and strong. I'm glad there is a lot of publicity lately surrounding the amount of chemicals used in cosmetics. That means that it is time to reevaluate what is going on with those products in your purses.

I approach this issue delicately as I know it is a sensitive subject for most women. Although we love to see our ladies made up and looking so very lovely – first and foremost, we want to keep you healthy! Once we become aware, it makes sense if we begin to take some steps to move away from known harmful thinks in all areas of our lives. So yes...this means you have to reconsider what's allowed in the makeup kit.

> *"ok...wait...I cut out the damn meat – but now I have to give up my lipgloss!?!"*
>
> —My cousin Kelly's comment on a facebook
> post about the chemicals in cosmetics.

I know that ladies are going to really flip out at the very thought of giving up that make up, especially the lip-gloss! But maybe we can reach a middle ground, find a healthy kind.

Remember our body is our temple.

This book is about beginning to monitor the overall amount of chemicals involved in our daily lives. Given all the disease of the western world, it is in our best interest to keep that number as low as possible. There are better alternatives that exist.

Lets take a look at some of the commercial chemicals that have become normal. From now on avoid at least some of these when you can. If powerful and creative ladies come together and have a small think tank – there can be new lines of healthy cosmetics coming from every social circle.

HOW DANGEROUS ARE OUR PRODUCTS?

"Consider this: propylene glycol is the main ingredient in antifreeze, yet go into your household cabinets and look at your toothpaste, underarm deodorant, shampoo, conditioner, lotions, soaps, or what have you and you will be amazed when you see propylene glycol. You will also see something called sodium lareth sulfate. Propylene glycol is everywhere, yet it gives you cancer! It is a colorless, vicious liquid used in antifreeze solutions and hydraulic fluids, paints and coatings, floor wax, pet food, tobacco products, and laundry detergents, but also cosmetics toothpastes, shampoos, deodorants, lotions, and processed foods. You will even find it in baby wipes. Check the labels, you will be amazed. This is why pets are getting more cancer than ever before. Pet companies are using it in pet food. This is why children are getting cancer at a higher rate than ever before. In addition to causing cancer, propylene glycol also causes dermatitis, kidney damage, and live abnormalities. It can cause skin rashes, dry skin, and skin damage. It is a major irritant to the skin. It also can cause nausea, headaches, vomiting, depression, and gastrointestinal disturbances. The other big problem with propylene glycol is that it doesn't leave your body. It stays in the tissues and continues to build up, causing more and more damage down the road. Keep in mind there has never been any long-range testing on the effects of these types of toxins used in various products."

Kevin Trudeau
More Natural Cures Volume 2

1. ## *Shampoo*
   Average # of chemicals: **15**

   The controversial:
   Sodium Lauryl Sulfate, Tetrasodium and Propylene Glycol.

   Possible Side Effects:
   Irritation, possible eye damage

2. ## *Hairspray*
   Average # of chemicals: **11**

The controversial:
   Octinoxate, Isophthalates

Possible Side Effects:
   Allergies, Irritation to the eyes, nose and throat; hormone disruption, linked to changes in cell structure

3. <u>*Eye Shadow*</u>

Chemicals: **26**

The controversial:
   Polytheylene terephthalate

Possible Side Effects:
   Linked to cancer; infertility; hormonal disruptions and damage to the body's organs.

4. <u>*Blush*</u>

Chemicals: **16**

The controversial:
   Ethylparabens – Methylparaben – Propylparaben

Possible Side Effects
   Rashes – Irritation – hormonal disruptions

5. <u>*Lipstick*</u>

Chemicals: **33**

The bullshit:
   Polymenthyl – methacrylate

Possible side effects:
   Links to cancer`

6. _Foundation_

Chemicals: **24**

The controversial:
> _Polymethyl methactylate_

Possible Side Effects:
> _Allergies – disrupts immune system – links to cancer_

7. _Deodorant_

Man, I remember spraying that freezing cold spray deodorant under my arms as a youth in Detroit! What the hell was that? There are many natural kinds to use instead, please explore them. Deodorant has a bunch of dangerous ingredients, it has always been linked with breast cancer.

Chemicals: **15**

The controversial:
> _Aluminum, Parabens, Propylene Glycol, Phthalates, Trisclosan, Isopropyl Myristate, 'Parfum'_

Possible side effects:
> _Irritation of skin, eyes and lungs – headaches – dizziness – respiratory problems_

8. _Nail Varnish_

The smell in a nail shop is strong as hell! I feel sorry for the people that are in that for hours at a time. I really can't stand seeing children up in there!

Chemicals: **31**

The controversial:
> _Phthalates_

Possible Side Effects:
> _Linked to fertility issues and problems developing babies(!!!)_

9. _Perfume_

Use sweet smelling essential oils instead.

Chemicals: **250!**

The controversial:
   Benzaldehyde

Possible Side Effects:
   Irritation to mouth, throat and eyes – nausea – linked to kidney damage

10. _Lotion_

Dump commercial lotions! Use Shea butter, Coconut or other oils instead! Propylene Glycol is the FIRST ingredient in some baby lotions. Smh. Incredible!

Chemicals: **32**

The controversial:
   Methylparaben – Propylparaben – Polyethylene Glycol (which is also found in oven cleaners.) -

Possible side effects:
   Rashes – Irritation – hormonal disruption

WHICH DANGEROUS COMMERCIAL INGREDIENTS SHOULD WE TRY TO AVOID?

It is not just the ladies that have to make some changes with the makeup; we all have to do some label reading. Please do some quick research about these ingredients. Attempt to avoid or at least limit the amount of these things that your family consumes. Even thought that will be difficult, that is going to help keep your family safe.

The sad truth is that ALL of these dangerous ingredients are actually not hiding at all. They are featured in MOST of the products at your local grocery store or commercial retailer. The only way to avoid them on any realistic level is to shop at different venues where the focus is on healthy products.

Trader Joes, for instance, has a variety of cookies, chips and cereals that mimic the look and taste of the commercial brands. Your kids will still be happy to get that as a treat because they are really sweet and sugary ~ just without HFCS and other chemicals of the commercial brands. We have to find alternatives like that.

As discussed in ELYGAD, making our own sauces and dressings is a great alternative. Remember that even if you are making an effort to eat healthier, commercial condiments and dressings are often full of sodium, artificial ingredients, colors and flavors. Whipping up your own will not only taste better – it will ensure that you are avoiding these dangerous ingredients listed below.

READ THE LABELS of all of the food products you give to your children. Google some of these for yourself so you can understand how dangerous these things could be.

1. Artificial Colors

Remember Red #40 and Blue #1, which are frequently used in the food products in the US grocery stores, is BANNED from use in the European Union due to their potential negative health effects.

Artificial colors are linked to: **Allergies**, **Sinus Congestion**, hyperactivity in children and increasing ADD symptoms.

2. Artificial Flavors

This general term could mean as many an 100 chemicals in combination. Artificial flavors have been known to cause **allergic reactions** and have been linked with **behavioral issues**.

Of course both of those are found heavily in products marketed to our children. Read those labels!

3. Artificial Sweeteners

Appear on labels listed as:
a. Sucralose
   i. Linked with Migraines and Intestinal Damage.

b. Aspartame (Equal, NutraSweet)
   i. Listen good: *3 out of 4* adverse food reactions reported to the FDA are from Aspartame! Many of the reactions are very serious including **seizures** and **death**! SMH.
   ii. Aspartame is **10% Methanol. Methanol** is a very deadly poison. It breaks down into formic acid and **formaldehyde** in the body.
   iii. Linked with **MULTIPLE** symptoms such as **headaches, birth defects** all the way to **multiple sclerosis**.

c. Neotame
   i. This is a brand new one, a cousin of Aspartame. It is largely untested, but soon we will no doubt find out some dangerous and deadly things about it too.

d. Acesulfame Potassium (Ace-K)

   i. Some researchers say it could be **cancer** causing. I'm not going to argue with them.

e. Saccharin (Sweet'N Low)

Our elders and people choosing these so-called "diet" products are ingesting too many of these! This sh*t is really dangerous – look it up for yourself. Don't focus on the fact that diet products might have less calories. Ignore that. All diet really means **MORE chemicals**; more BRAND NEW chemicals at that.

No thank you. It is best to stick with raw cane sugar, Agave nectar, Maple syrup or honey for sweeteners.

4. Trans Fats

Which appear on labels listed as:

*a. **Hydrogenated Oils***
*b. **Partially Hydrogenated Oils***
*c. **Shortening***

Trans Fats are very dangerous. They are closely linked to all of the big 3 American dis-eases: **Heart Disease**, **Cancer** and **Diabetes**.

This is another one that is only in America, it's banned in the European Union. It actually makes you more hungry leading to over eating and high rates of obesity.

5. Monosodium Glutamate

MSG is known to increase our appetite. It also is known to cause possible chest pain, heart palpations and/or headaches.

6. High Fructose Corn Syrup

HFCS is another one that is heavily used in America and banned in other countries. Anyone who saw my first book knows how I feel about High Fructose. American children eat it EVERY DAY, several times. Smdh.

7. Preservatives

These are things that commercial products include in order to make them last longer. These are things you want to avoid. ALL of them have a very sketchy track record.

*a. **TBHQ***
*b. **Polysorbates (60, 65 & 80)***

Products of Our Environment

c. **BHT/BHA**

d. ***Sodium Benzoate***

e. ***Sulfates***

These things are designed to preserve the food products so they last forever on the shelves, but they have the opposite effect on your body temple.

FOOD INDUSTRY MATHEMATICS

My problem with the current commercial food industry is that there is very little humanity involved in the entire process. It has gotten out of control. Things that are done mass production style in industrial environments that are so far from what we would do in our own homes and kitchens. **The larger the size of production the lower the quality standards fall.** The regulations must be fair to accommodate the enormous size of the operations and as consumers we lose in this scenario.

We can ignore things, but many of the products we know and enjoy daily come from these types of environments. All of our favorite breakfast cereals for instance, come from factories where **"100 Rat Hairs" is the acceptable level allowed per box.** That amount is generally regarded as safe. That is something we just have to accept as a part of the food system.

That is exactly why I try to keep away from chain restaurants and all commercial foods in general. They really don't give a damn and I don't want that madness to become part of my system.

100 Rat Hairs = perfectly acceptable

No commercial products for me man. That kind of stuff just doesn't add up in my book.

Label Reader II

Ok...go through your bathroom right now and take a look at the ingredients on some of the products you use everyday. Check out what's inside your lotions, soaps and other cosmetic products.

There is a natural tendency to simply trust the brands that we are accustomed to using. In the past, I never really paid too much attention to what was in the products I used everyday. I judged them mostly by how they smell and how they rub in or lather up. Or just stuck with the kinds that my family used growing up.

This is another area where you want to have some variety. Going to farmers markets, co-ops or health food stores, you can find some wonderful handmade soaps and lotions that smell good and feel great on your skin! Discovering local gems and unique items like that can be a highlight of traveling to different markets.

Now that I realize that the commercial products smell is really just a laboratory mix of synthetic chemicals – none of them smell good. It is not much different from the dangerous air fresheners. The smells come from the same laboratory.

Overall, there is just too much going on content wise for me to consider using commercial lotions. Check this out:

Popular Brand Lotion
Natural Aloe Vera & Cucumber

INGREDIENTS: WATER GLYCERIN, STEARIC ACID, GLYCOL STEARATE, ISOPROPYL PALMITATE, PETROLATUM, ALOE BARBADENSIS (ALOE VERA) LEAF JUICE, CUCUMIS SATIVUS (CUCUMBER) EXTRACT, HELIANTHUS ANNUUS (SUNFLOWER) SEED OIL OR GLYCINE SOJA (SOYBEAN) OIL, GLYCINE SOJA (SOYBEAN) STEROL, SODIUM STEAROYL-2-LACTYLATE, TOCOPHERYL ACETATE (VITAMIN E ACETATE), RETINYL PALMITATE (VITAMIN A PALMITATE), SODIUM ACRYLATE/ACRYLOYLDIMETHYL TAURATE COPOLYMER, DIMETHICONE, GLYCERYL STEARATE, CETYL ALCOHOL, LECITHIN, MINERAL WATER, SODIUM PCA, POTASSIUM LACTATE, LACTIC ACID, COLLAGEN AMINO ACIDS, UREA, FRAGRANCE, TRIETHANOLAMINE, DMDM HYDANTOIN, LODOPROPYNYL BUTYLCARBAMATE, DISODIUM EDTA, TITANIUM DIOXIDE (CI 77891).

WTF? Do you see why it is worth inspecting the bottles in your bedroom and bathroom?

You have to look at the small print because the front of the bottles have mostly beautiful pictures of nature. Like this one, which boasts about the naturally cool sensation of aloe and cucumber.

The bottom line is: ALL of the brands on the commercials, which are featured at all the common commercial retailers, are full of chemical ingredients. That is just the rule. Sometimes you may have to go through there and fish for the few exceptions, or pick the lesser of the evils – but you should know you are in dangerous corporate waters when you enter those megastores. Try to stay away!

Stick with simple, pure things for lotions like Shea Butter or Cocunut/ Natural oils. It makes sense that we to use natural things that the temple can recognize, those things go into your bloodstream. Add some real cucumber aloe juice to your own shea butter at the house. Be creative and make your own concoctions.

Popular Brand Body Wash

> INGREDIENTS: WATER, PETROLATUM, AMMONIUM LAURETH SULFATE, AMMONIUM LAURYL SULFATE, SODIUM LAUROAMPHOACETATE, LAURIC ACID, FRAGRANCE, TRIHYDROXYSTEARIN, SODIUM CHLORIDE, GUAR HYDROXYPROPYLTRIMONIUM CHLORIDE, CITRIC ACID, DMDM HYDANTION, SODIUM BENZOATE, DISODIUM EDTA, NIACINAMIDE*, PEG-14M, BUTYROSPERMUM PARKII (SHEA BUTTER) EXTRACT, TOCOPHERYL ACETATE**, RETINYL PALMITATE***.
>
> *VITAMIN B3, **VITAMIN E, ***VITAMIN A

Remember we wash every part of our body temple every single day. We should have some idea of exactly what is going to be running all over every curve of our sexy bodies on a daily basis. That is very up close and intimate.

Given the rising number of diseases and allergies that people get these days, it really does not make sense for us to use chemical based commercial products in our homes like that. Even if it is a little cheaper and conveniently stocked at the superstore, it can prove to be far too costly in the long run.

<u>The less chemical ingredients, the better it is for your system.</u>

Natural soaps are reasonably priced and in great variety. The natural oil soaps are great at home and easy to travel with. On the road or at the gym, it is easy to have your soap readily available.

It's very important to wash and maintain your body temple with simple and natural things as much as possible.

<u>Popular Brand Automatic Dishwasher Soap</u>

This brand does not disclose a full list of ingredients on the bottle. It does list their website – but I could not find an actual ingredient listing.

What the bottle does say very clearly is:

> First Aid Treatment: Contains sodium carbonate, sodium hydroxide, sodium silicate and chlorine bleach. If swallowed or gets in mouth, rinse mouth, give a glassful of water and call a Poison Control Center or doctor immediately.

This is the stuff we 'clean' our dishes with? It seems like these are far too harsh and strong chemicals to be used in our homes. Little things like that can add up in the long run. It's just as easy to get a natural brand, or make your own non-toxic version.

If something is toxic and dangerous in one way, it seems logical to assume it is dangerous in more ways than one. When a product for instance warns us that it is very toxic if swallowed — it seems safe to assume that we should not let that potent substance contacting your bare skin too! Even as we add it to hot water, the fumes of a product like that must not be too good for your respiratory system either!

LOCAL > commercial

Do this for me: The next time you are checking out at a huge supermarket/superstore, close your eyes for a brief moment and take a listen.

The chorus of hundreds of beeps at the same time can be nearly unbearable once you tune into it. Those beeps are an audible reminder of the corporate operation that is behind all of those items. It is essentially the heartbeat of the corporate system that lives and thrives off of our energy.

(And the beeps go on...)

Those products are generically mass-produced, preserved and shipped literally all over the globe. They carry stress along with them every single step of the way of their journey. It comes from the workers at the production factory, to the drivers of the delivery trucks, to the overnight stock people who display the stuff on the shelf, then finally to the beep drunk cashier that wishes you a routine 'nice' day.

You don't want to continue being next in line for those products. That is simply not the type of operation or items that you want to support going forward. That is not good enough for your body temple! You deserve more custom made shit.

Products of Our Environment

The chain retail (Walmart's) and drug stores (Walgreen's, Rite-Aid's, CVS's) that pop up everywhere have become the market place of a handful of huge corporations. Although there appears to be a wide variety, only a couple corporations own every single thing in there. There is only an illusion that we have a choice. To counter that we should begin reducing our dependency on commercial corporations and/or insisting on better quality products.

Just like you want to limit the amount of commercial food entering our bodies – our households should not be operating solely on commercial products and energy. Our own human energy should remain prevalent in our homes.

Pretend that those chain retail and superstores are not there. Start to form a smaller, more personal circle of products, services and people to support.

At least start chipping away at it.

Adopt new habits by making some items inside your home. Slowly but surely replace commercial items with your own proud homemade creations. Not only will that make you feel great, it will also take at least some financial support from the corporate pot. As consumers, we make statements and create changes with how we spend our dollars.

Going forward, look to deal more with smaller venues or people offering local products. We have to learn to be creative and work with people and stop running to the store for everything. Respect human craftsmanship and quality.

There are lots of people making wonderful products. If we start to seek that we will attract lots of new things to care for ourselves that we will love. Go to farmers markets, festivals and check the bulletin boards at the local healthy venues.

When you have hit the superstore out of habit and convenience – just grab your toilet paper, paper towel, q-tips and garbage bags and what not – then get up out of there.

We have to alter the way we operate in order to maintain a balanced lifestyle in our modern corporate-dominant society. **When you have to go to the gas stations try to *only* get gas. Leave the food, drinks and snacks alone!** It is not a food store. The only thing in there is corporate garbage food. Understand that before you walk in the door.

Products of Our Environment

Keep apples or nuts, water and a tea bag with you so the colorful, artificial rainbow of packages that surround you in every store or gas station will not be so tempting.

Farmers Market > gross-ery store

Learn to appreciate the human experience of a farmers market where you talk with actual people in the open air. No registers. No bar codes or beeps. Hand to hand contact with the same hands that grew your food. That is as direct as you can get without growing your own. Plus your produce can breathe, as opposed to being mummified wastefully in Styrofoam and plastic.

We should take a similar approach with the products we use in our homes. Our bodies are very intimate with the soaps and lotions that we use. Even what we wash our clothes and linens in warrants some serious consideration. Why not take a look at upgrading or making your own versions of some of those things?

Try to find and use some locally made brands that are not globally distributed. Remember to check the bulletin boards at your local health food stores to see what people are offering. Sometimes you will find people who left the corporate world and went into business on their own making products and soaps. Those are products you want to keep an eye out for and support. Consider learning to pickle and preserve foods for yourself too.

I know you may love the prices at the superstore, but learn to respect the quality of hand made items over generic commercial stuff. There is a great value in that which should be appreciated. It is comparable to the difference in a home cooked meal vs. TV dinners. A TV dinner may be cheap, but there is really no comparison. When I was growing up, fast food used to actually be decent. Now it is so artificial! That stuff is like plastic food now – it is below human standard.

We only have one body and one home to take care of. For most Americans it's true that the artificial colors and substances we use and that are in the processed foods we eat dominate our entire lives. That is a formula for disaster. Nature and humanity needs to always remain consistent threads in the fabric of our lives. Take this opportunity to readjust that balance.

Start looking for better products. Enjoy the creativity and uniqueness the handmade cosmetics. Your body deserves something special. Explore joining a local co-op where the products are selected with more scrutiny.

Forget that bottle neatly stocked in the superstore aisle next to the other commercial brands that is claiming to be the "the all new dry skin formula." No! **They machine make millions of bottles of that formula lotion for global distribution. They don't know a thing or care one bit about your skin.** Not as much you do! It would be so much better to find a local lotion that is made by someone in your circle with love and care. Find a brand where you can recognize ALL of the ingredients and stick with them. Alleviating products that contain possible cancer causing agents is a great place to start healthy skin care. And that is certainly worth a few extra dollars.

You can slowly educate yourself on the ingredients used in the products you like then make a custom blend of your own. It is cheaper and you save money that way. Who knows, maybe you eventually become the lotion lady in your circle. Farmers markets are perfect venues to support that type of grassroots business.

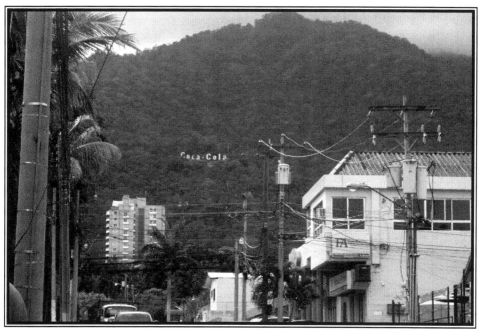

Nothing local about this: Nestled high up in the lush green mountains in San Pedro Sula, Honduras, it was hard for me to miss this huge 'Hollywood' style Coca-Cola sign. Not cool.

SUPPORT LOCAL ENTREPRENEURS OR BECOME ONE

After reading this book and doing some label reading around the house – we can clearly see how bad most commercial products have actually gotten. We discussed in ELYGAD how hard it is to live and eat outside of the corporate dominated food industry today.

For local producers of quality products there is a tremendous market. Whether we realize it or not, we are all in dire need of quality goods and services that we can trust again. The commercial products are no longer trust worthy – they should become a very last resort as opposed to our first option. The first option should be making things, or getting our things from those who do. The only ingredients we really can't get our hands on are the industrial things people want to avoid anyway. We'll have to make our cookies without the high fructose corn syrup and our lotion without the propylene glycol – that's perfect! That's the way it should be anyway.

There is a huge necessity for quality local goods and services everywhere. Most people are routinely using commercial products without a clue of the great dangers of doing so. That creates a huge market for the natural products. We all love our bodies and we should prefer spending our money within our circle than at a superstore. A small operation can be done with very little overhead costs. Maybe this is the time that we should consider starting our own small companies. Start getting out of that corporate job (that you can't stand going to because it stresses you out anyway), and go into business for yourself in some capacity. It will feel good doing something that will benefit people. Why not become the lotion lady or the salad dressing man in your circle as an extra hustle on the side?

Taking steps to produce some things and support local businesses are viable and tangible ways to start operating outside the corporate dominated world – at least on some level. We want to be prepared to survive outside of that web on page 32. In order to do that, our shopping habits have to change and that energy of production has to resonate within every community, especially in young people. Young children love to be involved in creating products. Instead of shopping all day on Saturday, spend a few hours making products with the whole family.

The Internet and social networks are making it increasingly easy to market and spread the word about our products or personal services. Resources like **YouTube, Kickstarter, GoFundMe** and other social media type outlets provide awesome new avenues for you to directly connect with people and even help fund your projects. We can advertise with the small, non-chain stores in your area. It can be lots of fun being your own boss and it can help fill a big need in this world.

Local products really enhance the character of an area and help to make each and every place unique. As consumers become more educated, we will come to appreciate that local hand made touch over commercial manufacturing. People are going to seek unique things, not keep settling for the same old mass-produced stuff that can be found literally everywhere.

Speaking of local production, **3D Printing** is a completely f*cking awesome technology that has been in development for over 30 years. Today 3D printing machines are small and affordable enough (starting in the $350 neighborhood) that this absolutely jaw-dropping technology is accessible to us all. Anyone could have the ability to be literally creating our own unique products from scratch. It's incredible! That allows us all the opportunity to instantly become designers, inventors and manufacturers. If you haven't heard much about 3D Printing do some research online – it is some futuristic stuff.

Check out some of the 3D Printing projects on Kickstarter or just get watch some videos online about it. The whole concept opens the door to endless possibilities.

It's hard to fathom that this really amazing stuff is out here but all the idiot box wants to show us is idiotic 'reality' shows and garbage like that. That just shows how much Hollywood is really aiming to keep people dumbed down and distracted. Our children need to be exposed to new technologies like this that will allow them to express their creativity.

D-I-Y

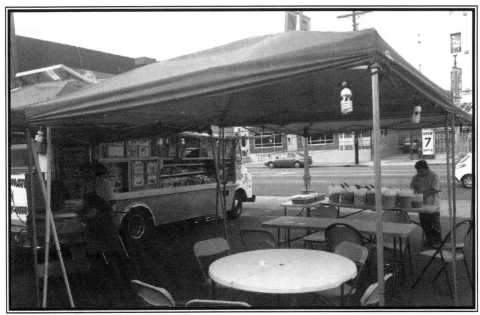

With the limited options in the urban areas it is time to start coming together and creating our own restaurants. Support people actually cooking real food. If you are one that can throw down in the kitchen, make some food and sell dinners to your people. It's better they buy that instead of that generic crap found at fast food or chain restaurants. Give them real food and keep that money circulating in the community. Sell dinners out of your car or the side door if you have to, that is where we have to take it. That is infinitely better than continuing to fatten the pockets of these major corporations who experiment on our families with their artificial, chemically laced food!

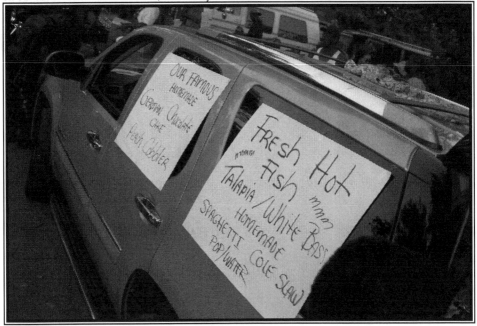

Products of Our Environment

"SEEK AND YE SHALL FIND"

Trust in the fact that you will attract the things and people you need simply by putting your focus there, because you are a Creator. I realize now in hindsight that I came across **Dr. Isis** years ago because she was exactly who I needed to be exposed to at the time.

I found out about Dhealthstore and the other resources listed here because it was exactly what I was looking for! That is simply the way the universe works. Walk your path and nature will supply exactly what you need. Embrace that.

In 2013 things continued to unfold incredibly for me. I got to meet and spend some time with two true walking legends that I have studied for years: **Dr. Sebi** *and* **Dick Gregory**! Whaa?

I also connected with two awesome homies from **Detroit** that are on the same page as I am: **Damien McSwine** and **Roi Meadows**. Everyone should get familiar with their work. Damien is an explosive author, powerful lecturer and teacher doing some really exciting work. Check him out online. I have to thank my boy Ottist for linking us up. It's just great to know that there are other real regular brothers out here trying to save our people! It's very motivating.

Roi is an incredible urban scientist who makes and patented his very own all-natural line of products, including this incredible soap he cleverly calls **D.O.A.P. Soap**. Connect with him on Facebook to learn more about all he does from shampoos to makeup without ANY chemicals. His stuff is 100% legit ~ no artificial ingredients. He might even hook you up if you tell him Ra 1 Pubs sent you.

Natural products like D.O.A.P. are safe and versatile. It can easily replace lots of other products by itself. It can be used as a body wash/scrub, applied as facemask, used as a shaving cream and as toothpaste! Something like that is not only saving your body from the toxins found in regular products, it saves you lots of money as well. How d.o.a.p. is that?

Natural things tend to be very versatile. Things like **Moringa** (pg 115) and **Black Seed** (pg 117) are things that literally everybody can benefit from using regularly. They are both good for absolutely everything. No side effects. A product like **Coconut oil** can be used a number of ways in eating/cooking, plus it is also great for the hair or as a lotion. **Essential oils** not only have great scents, they have many medicinal and cleansing qualities and can be used in many different ways. These are the types of things you want to begin to gravitate towards. The versatility makes it a worthy investment and they last a long time. The endless number of uses will also stimulate your creativity.

Between myself, Dejuty, Roi and a few others like my friend **Berjoh Fullilove** – I personally know the creator of nearly all of the cosmetics I use on my body, down to the toothpaste. I am just super proud of that! Some of the richest people in the world can't even make that claim! I hope people understand just how valuable that is today in America. The commercial products have only corporate energy behind them. There is no love or creativity involved with them. That has been replaced with cheap chemical ingredients.

I know the products that I use were created to be natural on purpose. Everything I use on my body is made with care, ingenuity, love and creativity. My people even want feedback about their products. They ask how I liked it and what I thought. They have a lot of care and concern for their creation. I appreciate that very much. That caring energy is exactly what we want to maintain our bodies with daily. That is another way to take health care into your own hands.

It cannot be said enough that the stores and pharmacies are filled with products that are very dangerous chemical mixtures. Remember not to be fooled by the words and pictures on the labels. They even put some garbage products in those healthy looking packages now. Don't be fooled by that. Read the ingredients. If it has any of the ones listed at the bottom of this page as controversial, put it back down. Why would we keep using that stuff?

I really hope that exploring the real dangers of these ingredients will lead you to make some changes right away. They have made it completely normal today in America for us to use a bunch of products that are made of mainly toxic sh*t.

PROPYLENE GLYCOL. PETROLATUM. SODIUM LAURYL SUFATES. PARABENS. BHA. BHT. MINERAL OIL. PETROLEUM. HYDROGENATED OILS. BROMINATED VEGETABLE OIL. GMO'S. OLESTRA. RED #40. BLUE #1 & #2. YELLOW #5 & #6. HFCS. HYDROQUINONE.

Be sure to look into some of those for yourself. This stuff is featured in most products at commercial retailers in America. And they know exactly what it does to people. We all know that if it is banned in other countries in the world, it must be for a damn good reason! So what does that say about our corporations and governing agencies? What do they think about us? How could we possibly continue to put any trust into this system or these products?

We can't.

Instead of raising the standards of American commercial products our government reacts to the imminent health problems in a different way. They take the opportunity to build more pharmacies and Dialysis centers in the hood. That, my friends, is American capitalism at it's finest. I encourage you to remove yourself from that ugly system. Yesterday.

In this Matrix where they obviously don't care, we are forced to be more proactive in taking our family's health into our own hands. There simply must be a change in the way we approach things. Steps must be taken. Wearing pink paraphernalia in October for breast cancer awareness is really cool and all but honestly, if you can try to stop the ladies in your circle from putting known dangerous stuff under their arms everyday that would seem to be a much more tangible means of prevention. Eating less animal products is proven way to reduce risks. That is the type of information you need to pass along to the beloved ladies in your life. It is time to become more aware and proactive.

Get outside of the box and seek some natural alternatives for your family. The resources you need are all around you. Even in your hands.

STAY ON THE PATH TO MAKING YOUR OWN PRODUCTS AT HOME OR GETTING LOCALLY HAND MADE PRODUCTS

This is a hard but necessary chapter. It is for information and not to discourage anyone at all. The most important thing is that you keep moving at your own personal speed, even if it's an inch at a time.

It is very important that we stay on the path towards creating more and more products at home. Try to remember to hold that as the ultimate goal. That is always, always, always the best option.

Don't get me wrong – it is really great that the local supermarkets are starting to have a little organic section. But remember that is _still_ the marketplace of the huge corporations.

A handful of corporations own basically all of the products that line the aisles of those commercial stores – even the good ones. The more we can learn to sustain ourselves outside the realm of those types of stores the better. That is the only way to be heard, to reduce our support of these mega corporations.

It is very hard to get around it. But remember that balance is an important part of the goal as well. Keep slowly shifting the scales until one day we are using more natural products and making more things at home than we are buying.

It is hard to get around the huge corporations these days – the supermarket is bought out. **Naked Juice is Pepsi. Odwalla Natural Juice is Coke. Tom's of Maine Natural Toothpaste is Colgate. Panera Bread is McDonalds.** That list goes on and on and on.

So even choosing the healthy options at the superstores still supports the wrong team. If it is your only choice, I would prefer to use Tom's of Maine rather than regular Colgate all day – but it is not your only choice by any means! Remember that the ultimate goal is maybe exploring making your own toothpaste – or finding someone locally (or online) who makes their own natural oral care products and supporting them. Decide you will stay away from regular commercial brands and you will see that many options exist.

Hell, Colgate does not need our little money anyway! A smaller business owner and their company would appreciate the business much more. You should feel good about supporting a growing business doing things the right way. The huge corporations could really care less about your support. I respect and appreciate quality – even at a higher cost. **We should expect to and be willing to pay a little more for well-crafted, higher quality products.** It also feels good to not be supporting this insane system.

Not to mention that our bodies are our Temples! (Make sure you get your wristband at ra1pubs.com and have a constant reminder!) We require high quality, natural products. Cheap commercial things are just not worthy fuel. We want to put in the highest octane available to make sure we keep running a very long time.

Water is a much better choice than a sugar-filled juice or soda. Buying an organic fruit smoothie, a fresh carrot/apple juice or making one of your own remains the best option.

Things that we make ourselves are far superior to any drink you can buy at a store because it is made just for you – with your own love and intentions. Bless your water and put your intentions into that as well. Stay home and blend up a 'moneymaking smoothie'. Create something that is exclusively yours and not available in stores.

There is simply no love left in today's commercial products. And far too often the only intention behind them is to keep us fat and hooked on those brands, artificial flavors and taste. Sadly, it is working.

If we remember to keep a water bottle and a couple herbal tea bags with us – it will save the money, plus keep us away from sugar filled and calorie packed commercial beverages. Empty calories from sugary drinks are where lots of the weight issues stem from in this country.

Let's take a look at an example of why it is important for us to keep pushing toward the ultimate goal of creating more of your own products.

Products of our Environment profile:

ALMOND MILK

Of course I personally recommend Almond Milk over Cow's Milk. Easy. It's a no-brainer.

But then in the next sentence I would recommend homemade Almond milk over the store bought kind just as easy.

Remember that this is not to discourage anyone at all. Replacing dairy milk with Almond milk on your shopping list is a tremendous upgrade. I'm thrilled to see my people taking my advice and trying that out. It is an important step.

The ultimate next step would be to make the Almond Milk at home (with your own love and intention of course ☺).

This might sound like a little too much hassle at first thought, but it is really easy! You can google it and make it right along with somebody on YouTube. ELYGAD has a really simple Almond Mylk recipe.

This is what I mean by us being products of our environment. We really need to change the ways we are used to operating. In this new age of information we must find ways to change along with the times. We cannot continue playing right into the hands of the faulty system.

A few of the hours that we'd normally spend out shopping at stores buying commercial products could be spent instead at home making a few products. I really encourage you to make that a habit. Try it. Use some of the recipes in this book or you can easily find some online. To make it more convenient, make large amounts of applicable things and freeze it. Have your homemade carrot/apple juices, soup broths, chili or homemade tomato sauces ready to thaw and use for convenience.

Back to our example of almond milk – the only ingredients required to make it at home are almonds, water and dates or vanilla extract. Maybe add a pinch of sea salt or raw sugar to your taste.

Let's compare that to the ingredients of a popular brand store bought Almond Milk:

> **INGREDIENTS:** ALMOND MILK (FILTERED WATER, ALMONDS) TRICALCIUM PHOSPHATE, SEA SALT, POTASSIUM CITRATE, CARRAGEENAN, SUNFLOWER LECITHIN, NATURAL FLAVORS, VITAMIN A PALMITATE, VITAMIN D2 AND D-ALPHA-TOCOPHEROL.

I wouldn't say that those are horrible ingredients by any means, especially in comparison to all the hormones, blood, puss, misery and suffering in a carton of cow's milk.

But at the same time it is quite notable how much more natural and simple the homemade version of it can be. Plus with the added ingredient of our own loving energy – we can dedicate and label that milk to do whatever we want. We can name it 'Wealth and Abundance Mylk' or whatever we feel we need it to be. That is the really awesome thing about creating at home.

As far as the commercial brand, **Carrageenan** is an emulsifying ingredient used in a great deal of commercial products – which raises a red flag. There are quite a few health concerns raised about it. The good thing today is it only takes a second to look it up online to form an opinion of our own. But you can see the clear advantage of using homemade versus commercial products, even with the healthy stuff.

Being truly proactive in your pursuit of health and natural things would involve trying to avoid those types of commercial ingredients. We definitely should seek to cut down the overall amount of commercial ingredients we use and ingest. Limiting and eliminating those things will allow us stay more firmly in control of our health.

Making more things at home will require some effort on our part. But considering the money that can be saved, the extra love that can be included and the commercial ingredients that will not be included – it is something that we should explore.

Working with family members, co-workers, neighbors or friends can make it more convenient. The next new moon, take on the project of making at least one thing for your household! Give it a unique name and purpose – tapping into your divine power of creation! ☺

I go into the store and use it like a library. Yes, some of the things in there seem to be way overpriced, but they all have a label with the ingredients printed on them in order of volume. Examine the things that you like and see what it would take for us to make our own similar version of it at home. You can make it even more suited for our specific needs and preferences.

This is the approach we must begin to take in order to sidestep the corporations.

Oh yeah, just to give you a little idea of how much the corporations have the grocery store and pharmacies have sh*t sewed up, check this out:

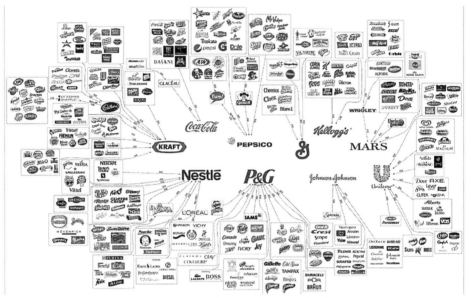

The only way to operate outside of that web is to seek local, natural products.
source: buzz.naturalnews.com
(I know that is small, check it out online to get a better picture.)

"…but if you want a bagel there are 23 flavors 'cause you have the illusion… you have the illusion of choice…there is no free choice in this country…"
— George Carlin

DEVELOP YOUR D-I-Y ARSENAL

These are some of the basic building blocks we can use to proudly begin producing our very own household items. We can use these affordable and versatile things in many different ways.

White Vinegar	Apple Cider Vinegar	Baking Soda
Coconut Oil	Aloe Vera Juice	Borax
Witch Hazel	Alcohol	Peroxide
Pure Castile Soap	Corn Starch	Lemon

ESSENTIAL OILS

Oils are a little more costly, but they last a long time and have a multitude of uses. There are far too many to list. Here a few that we might want to have in our collections. Add one every payday and soon you will have a powerful natural arsenal to work with.

Tea Tree Oil	Oregano Oil	Lavender Oil
Eucalyptus Oil	Peppermint Oil	Almond/Rose Oil
Geranium Oil	Orange Oil	Avocado Oil

Save your old containers of thing that you will not be purchasing anymore and rededicate them for storing our homemade products. It's a really good idea to have some Mason jars around for airtight storage as well.

If you are on fb, I highly recommend that you follow *'Herbs & Oils World'* and *'Learning New Skills for Survival'*; they both have incredible D-I-Y things that are really valuable. Invaluable resources.

DIY RECIPES

Here that we can start producing at home right away. A quick Internet search can provide ideas for homemade versions of nearly everything we need around the household.

Now it is time for a big mentality shift. We have to begin to think and operate differently. Producing things can save you money, time and gas from trips to the store – plus it is more natural and safer for your family. That is an old fashioned mentality that we need to reinstall today.

All Purpose Cleanser
- ♥ 2 cups of hot water
- ♥ 2 tablespoons of white vinegar
- ♥ 1/2 teaspoon of Borax (or baking soda)
- ♥ 1/2 teaspoon of Washing Soda Crystals
- ♥ 1/2 teaspoon Liquid Castile Soap
- ♥ 20 drops of Tea Tree Oil

Start with very warm water in a spray bottle and dissolve the Borax and washing crystals in the water by gently swishing it around. After they have dissolved, add the rest of the ingredients.

This soap is just as effective as any of those colorful cleansers with heavy chemical fragrances. It can clean almost anything very effectively. Get used to maintaining your home with simple things.

Homemade Bleach Alternative
- ♥ 1 1/2 cup 3% hydrogen peroxide
- ♥ 1/2 cup lemon juice
- ♥ 2 cups of distilled water (use equal amounts water/peroxide for stronger mix)
- ♥ 10 – 12 drops lemon essential oil

This mixture works well in place of bleach around the house and in the laundry without any danger involved. Just add all the ingredients into an old plastic bottle, simple. It is easy to make, plus very affordable and safe. It is not being extreme to make an effort to keep your household free of harsh chemicals – it's being proactive and smart.

Let go of the idea that bleach is needed to kill germs or whatever. According to Heinz, vinegar alone will kill approximately 99% of bacteria, 82% of mold, and 80% of germs when used for cleaning. Adding lemon or other things can make it very easy to make effective and safe household cleanser. We don't actually need chlorine bleach for anything.

Ridiculously Easy All-Purpose Citrus Cleanser
- ♥ A jar full of lemon/orange peels
- ♥ Distilled White Vinegar
- ♥ Distilled Water

Simply pour the vinegar into the jar until it covers the peels. Put the cap on tight and let the mixture sit for 2 weeks. After that, strain it into a spray bottle with an equal amount of distilled water. Shake and spray away. A simple, effective all purpose cleanser with a wonderful, natural (as opposed to a chemical), fragrance and zero chemical ingredients – **allergy**, **asthma**, **child** and **pet** friendly. It can do countertops, floors, windows, bathrooms, dashboards and more. Man…how simple is that? How affordable is that? It smells really good! Make your own unique label for it! Clean with your own products.

- A teaspoon of Baking soda could be added to the mix to give it a little more gritty scrubbing power.

Window Cleaner
- ♥ 2 cups water
- ♥ 2 tablespoons vinegar
- ♥ ½ tablespoon dish washing liquid

Pour two cups of distilled water in a spray bottle, add the other ingredients and softly swish around. And there it is! Simple, effective and non-toxic – I would encourage you to use a more natural, non-colorful brand dishwashing liquid.
(Distilled water is the best to use in these recipes.)

Air Freshener:
- ♥ 1 oz gin, vodka, or rubbing alcohol
- ♥ 6 oz filtered water
- ♥ 20 – 40 drops of an Essential oil of your choice: peppermint, almond, jasmine, lavender, rose or citrus oils all work well.

Listen, those commercial air fresheners are full of mystery chemicals. I don't trust those things at all! I get really upset when somebody sprays this stuff while I am even in the house! I need fair warning so I can GTFO. Seriously.

I cannot understand why we would spray that stuff in our homes where it will end up all in the carpets, clothing, sofas and linens. The babies, pets and plants don't need to absorb up all that crap! We aren't the least bit mindful to have proper ventilation while we excessively spray away, all over the house.

These brand new products with commercials proving they can cover up the smell of anything are simply too strong for our homes! I can't stress enough that if anyone in the house is dealing with asthma, sinuses, bronchial or allergy type symptoms how completely ridiculous it is to have this stuff floating around the house with them.

It is far more healthy and beneficial to simply burn (smudge) some sage, which actually cleanses the air and energy, or simply make your own safe and effective air cleaner. Burn some incense or essential oils for a natural fragrance as well.

Insect/Mosquito Repellant:
♥ 2 Tablespoons vodka/witch hazel/olive oil
♥ 10-25 drops of essential oil (cinnamon oil, lemon or regular eucalyptus, citronella, castor oil)

Make your mixture in a dark colored bottle and store away from direct heat if possible. Using several different essential oils can make the mixture more effective. It is safe to put on skin and clothes and can be reapplied every few hours.

I refuse to use a commercial insect repellant anymore. At some point I just knew I had to stop spraying that stuff all over my skin. That was back in the day, well before I had a complete lifestyle transition. I remember seeing the camp kids drench their skin with the latest, strongest chemical formula for repelling mosquitos. While that coat is still soaking in, some of the kids would then layer up with the latest commercial sunscreen product too!

In doing that we are in essence feeding our bloodstream a couple stiff chemical cocktails before we even sit down to pour cow's milk over the processed cereal with 100 Rat hairs in it! How this is NOT the Matrix? In the long run, that cannot be good for the body's defense system.

So I would definitely say that exploring some natural options is worth a try. It is so much better than smearing chemicals on our loved ones skin. Read those labels for yourself and think about it.

It's such a good idea to let the children get involved with creating their own products! All the way down to the label and artwork. That's a great project and it will also teach them to enjoy the creative process of making their own products. That will always give them an option other than the regular commercial stuff.

I know with this bug spray people will ask if it works. Well everyone I know that uses the sprays complain that they get bit anyway. With this one I know that I am not inviting chemicals in my bloodstream – and that's what works for me. Put your energy on it and make it work.

<u>Carpet Freshener</u>
- ♥ 1 cup baking soda
- ♥ 1 cup corn starch
- ♥ 15-20 drops of essential oil of your choice

Mix in a glass jar or airtight container. Before vacuuming, sprinkle on the carpet and leave it for 10 – 20 minutes then vacuum as usual. You can also sprinkle a little baking soda in the vacuum bag to reduce odors that might come from there.

For a light stain: Use an old toothbrush to brush a paste of baking soda and warm water into carpet. Vacuum the powder when it dries.

For heavier stains: Instead of warm water make the paste with baking soda and white vinegar and brush it in the carpet same way. It may take a couple of applications to completely remove the stain.

At least try these natural things first, before resorting to commercial products.

<u>Non-Petroleum Jelly</u>
1/8 cup grated beeswax (about 1 ounce)
1/2 cup Olive Oil

Combine beeswax and oil in a small saucepan. Melt over very low heat or in the top of a double boiler. Pour into a jar to cool and it will thicken into the jelly consistency that you might be used to. Look to avoid Petroleum based products going forward.

Homemade Toothpaste
- ♥ 3 Tbs Coconut Oil
- ♥ 3 Tbs Baking Soda
- ♥ 25 drops Peppermint Oil
- ♥ 1 packet of Stevia
- ♥ 2 tsp Vegetable Glycerine

Blend the Coconut Oil and Baking Soda together first, then add all the ingredients and mix into a paste. Store in an airtight jar – dip your toothbrush in and use anytime.

Homemade Mouthwash
- ♥ ½ cup of distilled water
- ♥ 1 cup of Aloe Vera Juice
- ♥ 2 tablespoons of baking soda
- ♥ 1 tablespoon Witch Hazel
- ♥ 20 drops of Essential of Peppermint

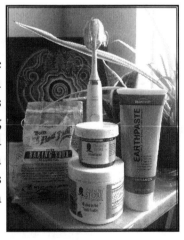

Non-toxic, homemade mouthwash! Mix these ingredients in Awesome. It is almost 10 damn dollars at the health food store for the brands I like at the health food store. The leading commercial brands are toxic as hell. We should not be putting that stuff in our mouths, or down our sinks. Making our own healthy mouthwash is an exciting and new project! A fresh, clean mouth without all the chemicals, have to love that.

Fluoride is very harmful and dangerous! Personally I either seek out natural brands of toothpaste that are fluoride-free, use them and dip the brush in my beloved **Healing Herbal Tooth Powder** from Dhealthstore – or just use **D.O.A.P.** soap by Roi Meadows it's the perfect blend! **Activated charcoal** is a great (chemical free) tooth whitener! **Food Grade Hydrogen Peroxide** and **Baking soda** are other affordable alternatives to the creepy commercial brands.

Hey, have you ever heard about:

OIL PULLING

Oil pulling is an ancient Ayurvedic (Indian) practice that dates back 5000 years ago or more. You take approximately 1 oz. of oil (organic sesame, sunflower work best), and swishing it around the mouth for 20 minutes before spitting it into the trashcan. You can start with 10 minutes and work your way up from there.

The oil collects and draws (pulls) toxins from the mouth, tongue and gums. The gums and tongue will noticeably begin to turn that healthy bright pink color. Through all the nerve endings in the mouth, the oil is said to actually pull toxins from throughout the entire body! It is important not to swallow the oil as it becomes filled with your collected bacteria. It turns an off white color by the end of your pulling session, some people might even see black specks in it. Yeah…ugh.

I was absolutely amazed to read about and discover the many health benefits from oil pulling (sometimes called Mouth Swishing). Put it like this, the people that practiced this never had a need for a dentist. Ever. So it is definitely something worth looking into. Swishing is another affordable, natural tool that we should try instead of expensive and painful dentist and doctor visits.

It sounds like an infomercial that in only 20 minutes a day, you can do some serious detoxing for the mouth and the entire body. Now how much would you pay? A bottle of organic sesame oil is less than 10 bucks. With healthcare the way it stands now, it is time that we look into ancient and proven methods that will allow us to take our family's healthcare into our own hands. Oil pulling is one of those methods. That is the premise of my next book so stay tuned!

Do some research about oil pulling online. Dhealthstore sells some mouth swishing oils that are lightly flavored, closer to what we might be used to. Always remember to try nature first.

"…oil pulling, or mouth swishing, performed on a regular basis, will leave your mouth fresher than any commercial mouthwash product on the market."
—Herbalist Dejuty Ma'at Ra

Homemade Deodorant

♥ ¹/₃ cup Coconut oil
♥ 2 Tbs Baking Soda
♥ ¹/₃ cup Arrow Root powder
♥ 10 – 15 drops of pure essential oil
(Essential oil of Cinnamon/Peppermint/Patchouli – etc.)

Mix the oil, baking soda and arrowroot in a small bowl. Mash it together with the spoon until you get a deodorant like, pasty consistency. Mix the essential oil of your choice and mix some more. Keep the paste in a small, recycled jar. Go caveman and dip to fingers in and rub it in the pits as you would with a commercial deodorant. Or you can use an empty commercial deodorant container and stuff it in there. It gets sloppy, but it can work.

Put your own creative label on there. Give it a minute to dry before putting on your fine linens.

Commercial deodorants have been linked with breast cancer for a long time. The underarm is a very sensitive area of the body. Here is an idea for a homemade version that you can put into a used named brand container. Look up the many noted dangers of these common commercial ingredients: **Aluminum, Parabens, Propylene Glycol, Phthalates** and **Triclosan**. See for yourself how harmful that sh*t is. Don't wear a pink ribbon for breast cancer – educate your family about this.

I can almost hear people asking, *'does it work?'* How well it works could be a good barometer for how clean or dirty your insides are. If you get ripe and funky – it might be time to try a full body detox or a colonic to clean the inside of your body. Things like oil pulling and drinking ample amounts of fresh water should keep our system detoxified so we won't sweat and smell like horses.

Give up the dead animals and clean your insides out – then see how much your body and stool odors drastically change.

Pipe/Drain Cleaner
- ♥ ½ cup Baking Soda
- ♥ ½ cup of Vinegar
- ♥ Large pot of boiling water

Have your vinegar ready while you sprinkle baking soda liberally down the drain liberally. Follow it with the vinegar. It will be fizzing away. When it stops then flush it a gallon or so of boiling hot water.

If you have a more major clog in your sink, use this mixture and let it stand for 3 hours. Then flush with hot water.

A mixture of equal parts vinegar, salt and baking soda may help open up a slow draining sink. Pour the solution down the drain, let it stay there for an hour and flush with boiling water.

Commercial Drain Cleaners are usually the most toxic substance in most households.

Cough Syrups
- ♥ ¼ cup of Apple Cider Vinegar
- ♥ ¼ cup of local raw honey

Pour mixture into a tightly sealed jar. Shake well before using. Take tablespoon every 4 hours or so. Label it and give it your own healing energy. There is no side effects or chemicals necessary to heal the body. Some people let a garlic clove soak in the mix as well.

TIPS AND TRICKS

☙ Sea Salt is a purifier. Similar to sage it can be used to **clear the air and absorb negative energy,** place a small bowl of it wherever you feel it may be needed, refer to your grid on page 97. **Clean your stones/crystals in sea salt** overnight to clear them.

☙ A soak with 26 to 52 ounces of sea salt in a hot bath is **great for muscle soreness** and is great for your body in general. Add 1 cup of Hydrogen Peroxide (or ¼ cup of 35% food grade hydrogen peroxide), for a very **healthy and therapeutic bath.**

☙ Spray your shower curtain liners with a spray bottle of vinegar once or twice weekly to **prevent soap scum build up and mildewing.** No need to rinse.

☙ **Loosen soap scum on shower walls or doors** with vinegar as well. Spray vinegar on the area and let it dry. Spray again and wipe clean.

☙ **Colored clothing that has become dulled can be brightened** by soaking it in 1 gallon of warm water and 1 cup vinegar – follow with a clear water rinse.

☙ Adding a ½ cup of vinegar to the rinse cycle will **eliminate static cling.**

☙ Apple Cider Vinegar makes a great **aftershave** splash. (or include it with some other ingredients!)

☙ **For healthy hair and to control dandruff:** Massage Apple Cider Vinegar into your scalp before shampooing.

☙ **For nighttime coughs, sprinkle your pillowcase with Apple Cider Vinegar** before bed.

☙ Be sure to brush after taking Apple Cider Vinegar or drink it through a straw because as it is abrasive to the enamel on the teeth.

☙ **Add a teaspoon of baking soda to your usual shampoo bottle** to help remove buildup from conditioners and other hair products.

- Add 4 tablespoons baking soda to 1-quart warm water, and soak feet for 10 minutes to **relieve foot itch.**

- Baking soda can and has long been used as both **toothpaste** and **deodorant**.

- **Activated charcoal** should be kept in every house in case of emergency. For cases of a drug overdose or accidental poisoning. If by chance one of those poison cleansers or cosmetics that I implore you to get rid of is swallowed. The charcoal binds with the toxin and prevents absorption into the intestines and stomach.

- Activated charcoal is a very safe and effective **tooth whitener**. Not only is it a non-chemical, it is also not abrasive to the gums.

- To make a quick and easy **face astringent** combine 1 cup of Witch Hazel with 2 tablespoons of alcohol (or ¼ cup of white vinegar). Use cotton balls to dip and rub it on the face.

- Straight Aloe Vera works as an **astringent** as well. Another **easy deep cleanser for the face** is cutting a lemon in half and rubbing it around your face before bed.

- **Clean your water bongs or pipes** with a simple mixture of rubbing alcohol and sea salt. Pour in the alcohol and then add salt and shake it up. The nasty residue will come right out.

- **Rue** is a unique smelling herb that can be found at farmers markets – among its many uses, it is good for **keeping pesky fruit flies** away. Get a bunch and put it in water in the kitchen.

- Ants/Spiders cannot stand the smell of **Peppermint** oil. Sprinkle some in a small open container in your kitchen – it **can replace those toxic ant traps** this summer. Ants don't like orange **or citrus peels** either.

- Periodically sprinkle the carpets with Baking Soda overnight and vacuum in the morning to **keep the carpet fresh and deodorized.**

- Rub the meat of a walnut over your wooden furniture to **cover up little nicks, scratches** and **dings.**

- A pinch of sugar or little maple syrup placed on the middle of the tongue will **stop a case of aggravating hiccups** immediately!

- Food Grade **Diatomaceous Earth** is a non-toxic substance that can help rid homes and pet areas of **fleas, ticks and other little mites like bed bugs.** Humans and pets can consume it internally as a natural form of parasite/colon/intestinal cleanse as well.

It's Raining Buckets

A simple yet great way to take advantage of what is free from nature is simply putting a bucket outside when it rains to catch water to feed the houseplants. Save some for a sunny day.

Just remembering to do simple, basic things like that can help to deprogram us from the product driven society. Plants love the acidic rainwater! That is more like their natural diet. It is great for them and it's completely free – like the all the best things in life. We want to keep our plants healthy because they can do the same for us.

Just like many of us don't like to drink tap water, our plants (or pets) don't want that regular tap water either! Get in the habit of at least letting it sit out at room temperature or sit out in the sun in order to release some of the toxins before watering the plants or feeding pets.

Our general approach to it all has to change. When someone is under the weather, the question we ask should not be 'what are you taking for it'. It should be 'what are you MAKING for it'.

...OUR DAILY BREAD

I always remember my friend Valentina telling me that in her family her mother baked ALL of the bread for their whole family. Period. It was a the regular occurrence in her household. She rarely, if ever had store bought bread at all. That always intrigued me. It makes so much sense.

Over the years people have complained about the rising costs of a loaf of bread. Making your own bread ends up costing much less, while you get to control the taste and all the ingredients.

Mom gets to constantly instill her loving and nurturing energy via that bread. **Every sandwich has her vibration in it. That is a natural form of health care.**

How cool would it be to have that wonderful smell of fresh bread baking right inside your crib? Delicious! That is the kind of thing that really makes a house a home.

As much as people complain about how expensive healthy food is, and rightfully so, we have to begin taking active steps like this to counteract that.

Here are the ingredients of a commercial loaf of wheat bread:

INGREDIENTS: ENRICHED **WHEAT FLOUR** [FLOUR, MALTED BARLEY FLOUR, REDUCED IRON, NIACIN, THIAMIN MONONITRATE (VITAMIN B1), RIBOFLAVIN (VITAMIN B2), FOLIC ACID], WATER, HIGH FRUCTOSE CORN SYRUP, YEAST, CELLULOSE FIBER, MODIFIED WHEAT STARCH, WHEAT GLUTEN, SOYBEAN OIL, SALT, CALCIUM SULFATE, CALCIUM PROPIONATE (PRESERVATIVE), SODIUM STEAROYL LACTYLATE, MONO- AND DIGLYCERIDES, GRAIN VINEGAR, MONOCALCIUM PHOSPHATE, CORNSTARCH, SOY LECITHIN, CITRIC ACID, DATEM, AZODICARBONAMIDE, POTASSIUM IODATE, **SOY FLOUR.**   R12-202

That says it all. It says way too much. The fact that a simple loaf of bread has all those ingredients cannot be ignored! That is not what we want to eat regularly. It does not say simple and healthy. It says chemically laced and ultimately deadly.

At home it is a COMPLETELY different thing. We get to control ALL of the ingredients and the ENERGY of that bread ourselves. **That homemade bread will not make us fat!** We won't be putting all those extra preservatives, dough conditioners or any of those other crazy ingredients inside it like the commercial stuff.

This has become a Facebook, Skype, e-mail and text me digital type of world. As much as possible, we need to hold on to anyways to consume things made with that family love. That is a form of nutrition that cannot be undervalued.

There ain't no love in all those Glycerides and Sulfates! There are allergic reactions and confusion for the body. That starts the increase of mucus and discomfort in the body. The meteoric rise in wheat and gluten allergies is not a coincidence at all. That is a result of the industrial farming industry and these genetically modified crops. Creating things at home is the way to ensure that it is good for you. We really have to realize the fact that they don't have decent food in the majority of American stores today and become our own producers.

If you cannot bake it, visit the local bakery where it is freshly made. Get that smell up in you. The big grocery stores have a little bakery section but often those ingredients are shady as well. Check for the day old items at local bakeries that are usually very affordable and still fresh. The healthy brands at stores cost a lot and they are still not always made with completely natural ingredients. Always seek better quality. If you cannot be the source – try to get things directly from the source.

This is yet another example of a product in which doing it yourself is the clear cut winner in taste, quality and value.

Your own family bread recipe is the type of thing you can try to establish and develop into a family tradition that your children and their children can continue to pass down. Our families will taste the warm love of home in that toast and that wonderful smell will always bring fond memories.

That is what I mean by living anti-corporation. In this day and age, we have to make sure the human element remains a consistent thread in the fabric of our lives. There is definitely something to be gained by doing some things the old fashioned (and even ancient) ways.

We can begin to restore health in this country in part by getting back into the mindset of creating and producing as opposed to always being consumers.

Select a few of the recipes in here and make something that you used to buy regularly. The money you save will help make healthy food more affordable too!

Check your local craigslist for equipment that can help make things easier for you to make your own products. Juicing machines, bread makers (you can use your oven), food processors, dehydrators, gardening equipment and more can be found at a great price.

There are also tons of detailed recipes online for homemade bread and everything else. Watch and see exactly how it is done on a YouTube video. Val's mom wouldn't give up her recipe for the book – it's become one of those old family secret recipe type of things. Apparently we have to create our own.

Actually…that's just what I'm hoping for.

KALE CHIPS

Kale is easily one of the most nutrient rich foods per calorie on this earth. It is a true super food, one that we want to keep in our regular diets as much as possible. It can be blended into smoothies, juiced, steamed, sautéed in stir-fries or eaten raw in delicious salads.

Dehydrated or baked Kale chips are really good and they are exponentially better for us than greasy, fattening potato chips. It is a totally different taste, but it is a crunchy snack that can handle a case of the munchies just the same. Kale chips also give us another perfect example of how doing it yourself is better and much more affordable.

I love Kale chips but they are so expensive. I've rarely seen them for under $5 a bag, sometimes they are even more than that. I don't even mind investing in something good for me at all, but that just seems way overpriced. Even though this text taught us how to cut some cost on household products – who the hell wants to pay 6 or 7 dollars for some damn chips?

But here's the thing, Kale chips can be really easy to make at home. Wash and dry it really well, then it can be slowly baked at a low temperature or oven poor man's dehydrated, (by heating them in the oven with door open). At a good farmers market a bunch of fresh Kale is only 1 or 2 dollars. That can yield at least 2 of bags of chips, if not more.

Sure it will take some trial and error before you learn to make them just how you like or buy them. If we just took one afternoon experimenting with various recipes, soon we will still be able to enjoy Kale chips at a fraction of the cost. It's actually really simple to do.

The ingredients are listed right on the package. Use that information along with some quick online research to emulate a brand that you enjoy. You can even customize the taste with spices to make it even more catered to your specific liking. Of course you make it with love – the clear advantage in creating things in your kitchen.

Keep in mind also that Kale and most varieties of greens are fairly easy to grow. Consider growing this superfood in your yard or window seal.

Maybe eventually if you are moved to, once you see how easy it is, you can sell Kale chips yourself at a lower price than the health food stores and generate a little business. Offer people around you, perhaps at your children's school or at your office, a healthier alternative to the norm.

That is the way I want you to progress. First you might want to bite the bullet and buy the high quality brands. Eventually you want to learn to make your own version of those brands, which will make it very affordable. Then share that knowledge with your circle. Work with those around you. That is how we can build new network of quality products to rely on.

A JUICE MACHINE IS A GREAT INVESTMENT

> *"If (we) keep eating laboratory creations as opposed to natures gifts – (we) will surely end up needing laboratory drugs and medicines."*
> —"Human Lab Rats" ELYGAD

I strongly encourage everyone to seriously think about investing in a juice machine and/or blender. Start making some of our own drinks at home. If we can inject that into our daily routines form time to time – even just once a week – it would be a tremendous upgrade for our overall health.

A super-size reason why Americans are consistently overweight is that we drink so many empty calories and sugars in the form of bottled juices, sports drinks and sodas. The orange juice that most of us enjoy every morning hardly even resembles the juice from real oranges! What is that stuff?

Make your own juice. Work with people in your circle. Maybe investing with a small group of friends/family/neighbors who want to improve their health could help make it more affordable. Create ways avoid the madness of commercial drinks.

If you don't have a machine (or if the cleanup is too much of a deterrent), consider making a weekly trip to the juice bar or Mediterranean restaurant so you can get at least one raw juice per week, that should be our minimum. If we make it a consistent part of our routine it can be viewed as a great form of preventative medicine. Drink some of your meals.

Juicing and making smoothies not only has many health benefits, it's also a lot of fun too. In this product driven world, the idea of 'making something of our own' alone is very exciting and hopefully contagious. The energy of DIY will naturally encourage us to branch out to making our own sauces and things like that too.

The wonderful smells and colors of the juices is intoxicating! The smell of fresh ginger, cucumber or cilantro filling your kitchen is an awesome benefit. Between the fast food restaurants pumping out those artificial smells and the artificially colored and fragranced products that line the shelves of our stores today – that natural smell in homemade juice production provides a very necessary balance.

Making fresh juice a part of our regular routine, in any capacity, is an absolutely <u>GREAT</u> way to reconnect with nature and get a quick boost for our immune systems.

A good strong blender will allow us to make our own delicious superfood smoothies. It encourages us to keep fresh fruit around which is always a good thing. Make sure to add your greens and any other natural supplements in and enjoy.

Keeping the stove off some days using fresh juices to replace meals is a sure and simple way to keep your weight down and your health up!

It also gives us a tool that can help us make our own medicinal mixes. Find out which fruits/veggies that are good for the specific condition of our loved ones and make fresh juices for them. Bottled juice, with its preservatives, processing and added sugars is not what we need when we are sick. We need real fresh juice – maybe then we won't even get sick. There is no comparison. And remember we get to put our own loving and healing energy into it.

We can even label it ourselves. Nothing can make you feel better than a homemade "Get Well Juice" – a kind that is not available in stores.

Plus homemade juice just tastes so fresh and great! Mixing apple in with anything is a good way to sweeten your juices. The best lemonade I have ever had is fresh-juiced apples with organic lemons (with the skin on). Pour that over ice and it is indescribably good! On top of tasting great, it is very healthy and uniquely different every single time! Then we can always use different types of apples to really tweak the flavor. Add ginger for a bite…whatever we want. That creation process can really become a fun adventure itself. Who wants to get the same exact (artificial) taste every time? How boring!

Juicing gives us a chance to give our bodies some much-needed natural nutrients. That is one powerful way to combat the processed food industry and keep nature prevalent in our world.

Investing in a good juice machine can help boost the health of everyone in our household. That makes it well worth it. Check on our website (www.ra1books.com) for advice about specific brands – but keep in mind that today there are tons of great products for all size households. Even for busy individuals on the go.

● Check out the work and life of Dr. Max Gerson.

● Listen to Dr. Thomas Lodi and his cancer centers and what they are able to achieve in great part with juicing and natural cures. Take a few minutes to check his videos online.

● See the documentary 'Fat, Sick and Nearly Dead' about the man who changed his whole life and cured himself of a rare disease through juicing.

● Remember to look on craigslist/ebay where you can often find items in new condition can be found for greatly discounted prices.

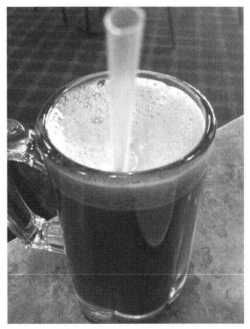

Fresh squeezed juice connects us with the essence of delicious nature!

NEW WORLD WATER

> *"…you gotta cook wit' it, bathe and clean wit' it – when it's hot summer time you fiend for it…it's what they dress wounds and treat diseases wit'… the rich, poor, black and white got a need for it…consumption promotes health and easiness…American's wasting it on some leisure shit…Other nations be desperately seeking it…"*
>
> "New World Water"
> Yasiin Bey (Mos Def)

Water is vital to life and health on every level. Each one of the millions of cells in the body needs water to function properly. Keeping hydrated is a must. ALL living things must have water to survive.

Ideally we should be drinking ½ **of our body weight in ounces** – everyday; either that or go with the familiar '**8 glasses a day**' slogan that we all grew up with.

Most of us are falling short of that on a daily basis. That is a lot of water! I created '**Water Wednesday's** as a weekly reminder to get full hydration at least once per week. That is a good habit that will 'spill over' into the rest of the week.

Drinking water is not the only way to hydrate the body. Raw fruits and vegetables are composed of mainly water and are a great water source. Eating lots of raw foods will keep us loose and hydrated. Make some fruit and water days where you eat very light, give the digestive system a break and drink some good water.

Although every beverage is made up of mostly water – the amount of sugars, sodium and/or caffeine contents in bottled drinks can make the body retain water (sodium) or even decrease water levels (caffeine). Many nutritionists and health professionals suggest that most humans are walking around drastically dehydrated.

We can all be in agreement that drinking water is very important. I think the question (something that I get asked an awful lot), is **what type of water** should we be drinking. I don't know that there is really a definitive answer for that question. I think we should be drinking the best water available to us. Let's take a look at some of the different types of waters on the market and some of the options we have today.

First of all, no matter what type of water we drink, we should be mindful to...

DRINK RESPONSIBLY

It is hard to believe that water of all things has become an 800 billion dollar industry. **The amount of plastic that we use and waste daily is a huge problem for our environment** all by itself. The cases of small plastic bottles may be convenient but it forces us to use and throw away literally tons of little plastic bottles over time. We don't want to add to the destruction of our planet! It is a really great idea to invest in a good reusable (plastic, glass or stainless steel) water bottle to use daily. Make it a regular accessory like your purse or phone.

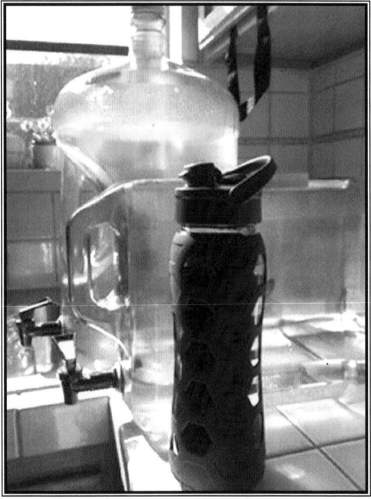

Using large refillable containers and refilling our own reusable bottles is a more earth friendly way to drink water. **A water bottle reminds you to drink water and it's the perfect way to monitor your daily water intake.**

Here is a look at some different kinds of water/aqua/maji/maa'/l'eau/wasser:

ALKALINE WATER

Alkaline water is the Cadillac of waters.

An acidic body is unhealthy. As **Dr. Sebi** teaches, everything that is a pure product of nature (God) is Alkaline. Alkaline water helps increase the body's pH level while completely hydrating the body. It can help to hydrate and drive out acidic toxins all the way down to the cellular level. Because it is ionized (or micro clustered), meaning it has a different molecular structure, it is said to be up to six times more hydrating than regular water. The smaller cluster of cells allows alkaline water to be more easily absorbed into your body's cells.

I know many people who love and have become absolutely committed to drinking alkaline water. There are many reported benefits ranging from glowing skin, increased energy and even a sensation of lubrication all the way in the joints and muscles. Although there may be some scamming companies, be clear that alkaline water itself is *not* a scam by any means.

Try some out with your family. For many people switching to alkaline water turns out to be a gateway to an overall healthier lifestyle. It can be the start of many changes. Dispensaries that sell alkaline water generally attract a special brand of people who are really enthusiastic about wanting to feel better. It's a great atmosphere.

Ideally, you would like to use alkaline water for all of your daily kitchen needs like making teas, soups or rice. A couple 5-gallon spigot refillables at the house in constant rotation could be just what the naturopathic doctor ordered. Passing by it at the house all the time encourages you to drink more water. Seeing how important water is to our daily lives and how much of it we use, an alkaline water machine is a very worthy investment.

While they can be pricey, there are tons of models available today ranging from 200 to 2,500 or even more – it is a very logical long term investment seeing how important good water is to health. Check the local craigslist for a good deal. Maybe you can start a very small business operation and let your people spend the money with you instead of giving it to stores to help offset the cost. Everyone, without exception, needs access to good water. Thinking of creative ways to generate some income while truly helping people at the same time is a sure stream to success.

ACIDIC WATER

There is not enough mentioned about the uses of Acidic Water. It is usually available where we get alkaline water. It is **not for drinking** but it has tons of uses and can actually replace a lot of products in our home.

Acidic water is great for the skin and can help with acne conditions. It can be used as an aftershave or as a hair rinse after shampooing. It is good for dandruff, itching and protects the hair.

It's a natural disinfectant, perfect to use as a vegetable wash and for washing meats (if applicable), it can help prevent the spread of e-coli and other bacteria. Cutting boards, counters and sinks can be non-toxically sterilized with it as well. It can be used in place of bleach to help whiten clothes. It can even be used for brushing, it helps to both prevent plaque and whiten teeth.

It is also great for promoting growth in our houseplants – rainwater is naturally acidic as well. The alkaline water machines produce the useful acidic waters as well. That makes it an even more of a versatile and money saving investment.

DISTILLED WATER

Water is something that you really have to experiment with and research on your own. I had always been taught that distilled water was good for fasting or detoxing, but not so much as our regular drinking water. Distilled water is best to use in our homemade products and good for cooking.

I learned that the vibrant and very beautiful 70 plus-year-old raw foodist Annette Larkins from Florida drinks a gallon of distilled water daily. She also grows all of her own food and catches rainwater to drink and water her garden with. She distills her water herself too. That is the next level! Doing it yourself is always the best option. She is my idol.

> *The fluoride in our municipal water comes from hydrofluorisilicic acid, a toxic waste from industry. This has NEVER ONCE been tested for safety. It's banned in 98% of Europe.*
>
> —The Fluoride Deception

SPRING WATER

The most popular bottled water is probably spring water. It taste much better than tap water. After some head spinning research, I am really going to step my water game up from now on. If I don't have alkaline water, I generally look for the best spring water option available.

I won't name specific brands in here, but I guess people have their favorites. The huge soda companies that jumped into the water business – I proudly choose to avoid those brands. POE is all about considering what we are supporting on a larger scale when we buy our products. I want us all to become more well-informed and responsible consumers.

"Every day America's largest bottled water corporations Nestle, Coke and Pepsi pump millions of gallons of water from the earth, bottle it, ship it and sell it back for 1900 times the cost of tap water…"

~ A great water documentary "Tapped"

It is worth noting that any company bottling and selling water within a state, like most of them do, are basically unregulated. Just because water is in a bottle, it does not mean it is pure. That stuff could very well be full of toxic waste too.

TAP WATER

Remember before the whole bottled water craze started? We all grew up drinking water out of the sink. My favorite water growing up without question was in the backyard out of the hose…it had that little summertime hose taste on it. Delicious. There is an ongoing debate if bottled water is actually any better.

Coming from Michigan, I have friends on both sides of the tap water fence and I understand that. The whole water thing is very confusing. Personally I try to avoid drinking unfiltered tap water in general. I'm a hippie though, and all the hippies drink tap water no problem. So at times I will refill my bottle with tap water in certain regions of the country or at a certain level of thirst. I usually hook my water up with some of my own minerals or herbs that are always in my backpack. I prefer to cook and make tea with clean water when I can, but I will use tap water for that too without fretting too much about it. Stressing about anything is usually worse for us than what it is, so whatever I do I try not to be stressed about it.

There are some very good questions raised about the integrity of this water industry – like how do we know that the bottled water is not just tap water anyway? That is a very good question because **as many as 40% of water companies were found to be merely bottling tap water.** It has become a billion-dollar industry today and many companies 'spring up' to take advantage. We don't want to be foolish and buy the same stuff we can get from our sinks.

Another argument for drinking tap water is that we generally shower, brush our teeth and cook with that same tap water daily and it doesn't hurt us – so why not drink it? That viewpoint certainly holds some water as well. The skin is a huge, absorbent organ and the warm shower opens our pours for that chlorinated water. Our ice at home is usually made with tap water too. So unless we put filters on our entire home or at least the showerheads – which is actually a great idea – it is very hard to get around the reality of tap water being a part of our life in some capacity.

In the good old days the dangers of municipal water was not really a concern – or at least not like today. The EPA suggests that there are **as many as 90 contaminants in tap water, headlined by chlorine and fluoride.** Local water departments are required to provide a detailed report on the tap water content found online. (*By contrast, bottled water companies are not required to submit their reports to anyone or display them publicly.*)

It is very much worth noting that the whole fluoride thing is completely horrifying. It has always been promoted as healthy for children's bones and teeth – but we also know a toddler could die from ingesting too much of it! The use of fluoride is banned in Japan and most of Europe.

The fluoride that is added to our municipal water supply is literally a classified toxic byproduct of fertilizer, aluminum and nuclear weapon production. The poison is barreled and sent unrefined to municipal water treatment facilities around the country. They did some quick Matrix stuff and created a huge ad campaign promoting fluoride as healthy! Now they are allowed to use our public drinking water to dump these dangerous chemicals.

Historically the Nazi concentration camps used fluoride to keep the inmates passive. It is known to impair the function of the brain and pineal gland, lower IQ levels in children, impair learning and it has been linked to cancers. Yet a Federal mandate ensures that it is added to the water supply of over 70% of US cities. WTF? The land of the free huh?

We should be well aware that homemade water filters is an option to consider exploring. Purifying water through **rocks, sand** and **charcoal** is the age-old natural way. Remember this is the time that we are looking into different ways of operating at home and becoming less dependent. There is a natural way to produce everything we buy. Always be mindful of that.

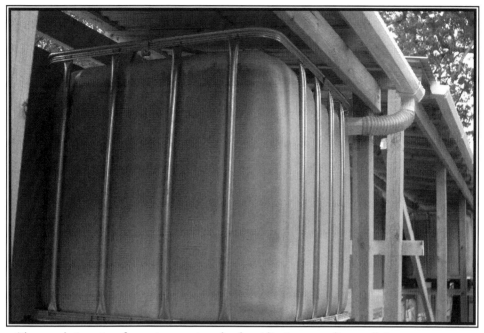

The cumulative price of water is expensive – but humidity is surrounding us all time.
Sometimes it even falls from the sky for free!

Drinking really good water is like having a brand new pair of good shoes on. Yeah… you can grab a cheap pair of shoes but there is just something about the quality and feel of rocking some high quality kicks that is unmistakable. It makes you strut a little differently. It's the same way with water. Knowing that you have upgraded and are drinking a better quality, clean water makes you feel good about yourself! Every time you refill your water bottle you are doing something awesome for your temple. You are consciously not adding to the plastic problem that is destroying the planet – that is definitely something to strut about.

TREATING/ENHANCING/CREATING OUR OWN WATER

Do what you can to make your drinking water as good as possible. It is something that we should always look to gradually improve, like everything else in a health journey. Water is a very important component of health.

Boiling tap water to purify it is certainly not a bad idea…but be aware that boiling it is by no means a cure all. It is effective for some things but it does not kill all of the chemicals and contaminants of water. Some even suggests that boiling tap water only brings some the unwanted content right up to the surface. I would reason that it is still better than nothing.

It is also not a bad idea to pour tap water and **let it sit for ½ hour or so to at least let some of the unwanted gasses evaporate** before drinking it. Let the container of water sit in the sunlight for a spell before feeding it to plants or pets too.

A pitcher with a quality filter is another way to improve our tap water. There is an awful lot of crap we are trying to eliminate, but some form of filtering is certainly better than none. Even **portable water bottles have decent filters** built in so we can fill up anywhere on the go and ultimately save lots of money. It's perfect for a traveling lifestyle, in places like airports or at other public events.

Other creative ways can be found to enhance your water. **Adding lemon** to water is said to be like the poor mans alkaline water. Dr. Isis taught me to cut organic lemons in quarters and keep them with me in a glass container to fill up during summer excursions. That is a form of filtering too. It is also said that **wheat grass** can be used with tap water to help neutralize the effects of fluoride and other potentially harmful water ingredients. Fill your pitcher and let it sit with a handful of fresh wheatgrass. Always remember that you have the ability to **place your own energy and intention** in your water. Take the time and do that no matter what kind of water you're drinking.

The monoculture system of industrial farming is ravaging the topsoil leaving it depleted of minerals. Ionic minerals (**zinc, copper, selenium**, etc.) can be added to water periodically to supplement those very important minerals. **Herbs** and **herbal teas** can provide a lot of our necessary nutrients as well. Explore some the many **liquid herbal extracts** that can be added to water that we drink to help bolster the benefit and quality of it. That's a fast and easy way to proactively give our immune system some support.

Alkaline drops can conveniently be added to any beverage, (water, coffee, wine, beer, etc.) – to help raise it toward alkaline range. When your watching the game with a cold local beer, don't hesitate to put some alkaline or zinc in there too.

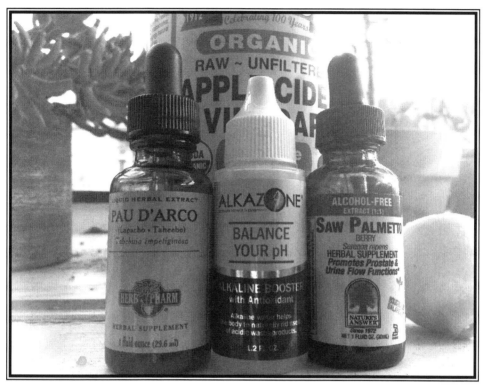

These are the kind of extra weapons that we can use to keep our immune systems strong.

FILTERING OPTIONS

The only way around the corporations is to be proactive and take steps to make the water you drink better. Work within your means and try to get water as pure as you can. So many different types of systems are available. Start with something and gradually improve on it. The ultimate solution might be investing in a **home filtering system** which ensures that every glass of water, hot shower, bowl of soup, ice cube, cup of tea, every dishwasher and washing machine use will be with clean quality water. That can really make a serious difference over the years. It is a worthy investment because everyone in the household benefits from that, even the pets and plants. Plus it saves the money of needing to buy bottled water.

A water softening system for the shower, drinking water, washing machine or for the whole house is another option worth exploring. All of this can be a part of creating a safe place in your home. Soft water can largely extend the life of the plumbing and appliances at the house. Plus it works much better with the natural soaps and products we are all going to be using from now on. A shower filter that will at least remove chlorine (bleach) out of the water makes perfect sense and it's an affordable step to take. Showering in water without chlorine and heavy metals day in and day out has to be so much better for our skin and hair – and the environment as a whole. I'm in!

TAP INTO A TRUSTED SOURCE

Just like with food and products, it is ideal today is to know more about the source of your water going forward. The industry of unregulated bottled waters and the massive problem of plastic container waste is threatening the health of our entire planet. It is very serious. It's time to turn the page from that. Get water from a local water store where you know more about the processing of the water. They generally offer flexible delivery schedules that make it convenient if you choose that route for your home or office.

The awesome **air water systems** are great water production systems on the market for the home or office. They actually extract water from humidity in the air and filters it into clean drinking water. There is no plumbing necessary. Just plug it in and drink up. It could be the end of buying plastic bottles of water. The idea of extracting water from thin air…how incredible! It is much better to invest in something like that as opposed to buying and throwing away cases of plastic bottles every week from the supermarket. It is time to evolve from that.

An **Ionizing Alkaline water machine** or **reverse Osmosis system** are investments worth looking into as well. We are paying a lot of money for water on a regular basis. It's a very ideal situation to be able to produce better quality, clean water right at the house. After the initial investment you will always have access to good water. It's going to be a valued amenity moving forward.

I always remind people that if several households or neighbors chipped in and bought an ionizing water machine it would quickly pay for itself with the money saved. Each household would be producing drastically less plastic waste over time and everyone would be drinking great water. Remember the acidic water is great for household and cosmetic uses. A group of family members, friends, elders, athletes or co-workers could work together to make it affordable and convenient. At this point, we all basically have the same needs and coming together makes it much easier to address them.

Different types of **homemade water filtering systems** or **rain collection** systems are not rocket science to set up. All types of set ups and methods can be learned for free at the fabulous YouTube University. I would encourage young men and women to spend some time honing survival skills like that. That could be a good hustle for you while offering a very valuable service to people in the community.

IT ALL BOILS DOWN TO THIS:

Our planet is begging us to stop wasting so many plastic bottles.

On one hand we have **tap water**, which is regulated by the EPA. It must go through certain amounts of monthly testing and detailed reports of the results are made available to the public. That is the good part, I suppose. The bad part is if you look at that report it is pretty much horrific. Think about all the human waste and shit that goes down the drain in a city – it is hard to purify that

On the other hand you have **bottled water**, which falls under the jurisdiction of the hands off FDA, they leave it up to the companies to conduct their own private testing. They don't have to tell the public anything. So who knows what is actually in bottled water? It's not enough to fret that companies are just taking our local water and selling it right back to us for huge profit – they could actually be using bottled water as a dump off for toxic chemical wastes. If you haven't noticed, that's the way they get down in the Matrix. Just because water is packaged in a bottle doesn't mean it is clean or safe. Look for some indication about the purification process used on the label, like "reverse osmosis". Do some light research on the companies and try to avoid the major commercial brands.

You can upgrade your water in some capacity. Find a water dispensary in your area. A new water source, a shower filter, a new refillable bottle or a kitchen sink filtering system could equal a major boost in your overall health and energy for the whole family. Exploring creative ways to make filters or utilize **crystals**, **magnets** or **the sun** to purify water can be valuable skills. Always remember to put your own great energy into whatever water you drink before it enters your temple. Use and drink the best quality water that you can.

And please remember that **our planet is begging us to not waste so many plastic bottles** – we can't ignore that.

IGNORANCE IS BLISS

> *"People are fed by the food industry, which pays no attention to health, and are treated by the health industry, which pays no attention to food."*
> —Wendell Berry

The truth can be hard to swallow sometimes, both literally and figuratively.

Who really wants to have a deep discussion about the bloody truth of exactly where their meat comes from – especially while their eating it? Nobody.

The food industry's pictures, commercials, propaganda and packages have created the illusion that this is the still the same old-fashioned food that we used to know. We are almost inherently lulled into the sense of security that comes along with familiarity.

We'd like to assume that the values and integrity of the food industry have remained in tact, when the truth is they have not. In order to stay comfortable (and sane), we continue to consume the illusion right along with processed foods. Things are easy to ignore.

We can eat things that taste good even with a fairly clear understanding that it might not actually BE good.

I know from experience that it's really easy to totally block out the whole slaughterhouse thing and simply enjoy the hamburger.

It is the American way. Ignorance is bliss.

It smells and tastes good once its all seasoned and cooked – but how tortured was that animal? How filthy was the overcrowded environment? How many hormones, steroids and anti-biotics have those sickly animals we eat been treated with? The truth is you probably don't want to know! I feel you. It would ruin your appetite.

We are really good at keeping the blinders on and have taught ourselves to not even deal with that aspect of it. Collectively we have chosen to be willfully ignorant and just enjoy the taste.

Eat the cake Annie Mae!

> Cypher: *You know...I know this steak doesn't exist. I know that when I put it in my mouth, the Matrix is telling my brain that it is juicy and delicious. After 9 years you know what I realize?*
>
> [Takes a bite of steak]
>
> Cypher: *Ignorance is bliss.*

In conjunction with the artificial foods we consume – perhaps as a result of the food – we have developed an **appetite for illusions.**

The corporations and advertisers sell us illusions and low quality, genetically engineered food like products. And we faithfully not only accept it, we also support it.

The advertisement says, "try our all new crispy chicken made with 100% white breast meat." I KNOW that people must realize how skeptical that is.

But, I will be damned if people aren't lined up the next day ordering the hell out of that new crap. Through marketing, advertising and tell-lie-vision – they have us completely hooked on that "food".

In fact we are hooked on illusions and basically trained by the marketing and media machine in general. My theory on it is this: *if you eat the bullshit they feed you, then you will eat the bullshit they feed you.*

They know that if we are able to fool and blind our own selves into not only accepting but also actually craving synthetic food – and feeding it to our children – we will be susceptible to accepting all the other lies America feeds us. We allow them to feed that bullshit to our children too.

They feed us all of these phony politics quite easily too. All kinds of lies are served up through mass media, through religion, education and history – and they already know Americans will eat it. Hell...we buy and eat illusions all day, everyday. Billions served.

So they continue to feed us lies about the danger of terrorism for instance.

They convince us that we need to have war in order to restore peace. They serve up lots of little bullshit like that and we eat it. Conspiracy is real.

They start planting false seeds and train our minds early in our lives. My nephew Chase at only a stuttering 4 years old told me that he knows for sure that Columbus discovered America! The United States is a corporation that was established completely on lies and illusions.

A fast food company is the main sponsor for the Olympic games as if all these world-class athletes could fuel their bodies with meals from there. We know that can't be so. But they put the illusions in our faces – and we eat it up.

Surely our willingness to consume artificial foods is part of the reason that they are confident that they can control and manipulate the minds of the people. **Consuming processed foods does not support natural thought process or body function.** All commercial snacks are machine made (blue pill) food that suppresses our natural human instincts, while natural whole foods awaken us. Living food that is fresh out of the earth contain the wisdom and intricacy of nature inside it.

That living food is our direct connection with nature. That connection feeds our souls. Too many of our souls today are starving due to us living off of these process foods.

Our society has become so product driven, we are losing our connection because we are eating too much out of boxes, packages and bags – and not enough things out of the ground. It is out of balance. This used to be a nation of farmers; family dinners used to be a very important part of our lives. Now it is a nation of consumers. We are literally letting the corporations feed us.

If we paid any attention we would see that the FDA has many close ties with Monsanto and the genetically modified food movement. They do this shit right in our faces, blatantly! Like President Obama appointing **Michael R. Taylor to the position of Senior Advisor to the Commissioner of the FDA. He was former Vice President and heavy lobbyist for Monsanto,** (educate yourself on that.) The bottom line is the government agencies are not protecting our best interest anymore – **they are experimenting on us** in real-time and playing monopoly along with huge corporations.

We continue to be more than willing subjects in their experiments. We pay to be the subjects. I know people see all those crazy negative posts about fast foods, but for some reason we will keep pulling through the damn drive thru for the latest sandwich.

Only our willingness to do things differently can combat the food industry today. We have to be aware and only deal with high quality things going inside our body temples. Resorting back to old-fashioned ways of doing things is not a bad idea at all. Connecting with an old fashioned family farmer is just a matter of getting online and reaching out. Our local grocer is not the only option.

It is important that we wake up and realize the game.

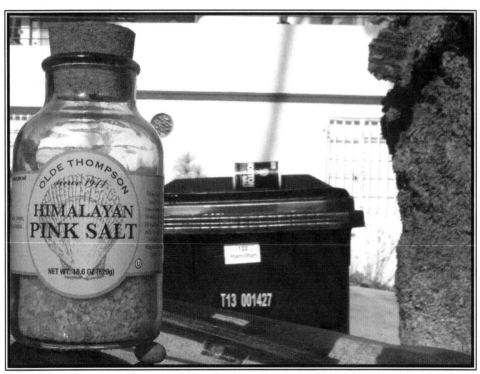

Trash that white table salt!!! A good quality colorful Himalayan Pink or Hawaiian Black sea salt is an easy and almost mandatory replacement for white table salt.

MOOR FOOD INDUSTRY MATHEMATICS

Amyl acetate, amyl butyrate, amyl valerate, anethol, anisyl formate, benzyl acetate, benzyl isobutyrate, butyric acid, cinnamyl isobutyrate, cinnamyl valerate, cognac essential oil, diacetyl, dipropyl ketone, ethyl acetate, ethyl amyl ketone, ethyl butyrate, ethyl cinnamate, ethyl heptanoate, ethyl heptylate, ethyl lactate, ethyl methylphenylglycidate, ethyl nitrate, ethyl propionate, ethyl valerate, heliotropin, hydroxyphenyl-2-butanone (10 percent solution in alcohol), a-ionone, isobutyl anthranilate, isobutyl butyrate, lemon essential oil, maltol, 4-methylacetophenone, methyl anthranilate, methyl benzoate, methyl cinnamate, methyl heptine carbonate, methyl naphthyl ketone, methyl salicylate, mint essential oil, neroli essential oil, nerolin, neryl isobutyrate, orris butter, phenethyl alcohol, rose, rum ether, g-undecalactone, vanillin, and solvent.

=

"*Natural*" Strawberry Flavor

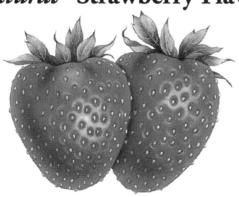

Products of Our Environment

GET IN TOUCH WITH NATURE

> *"Overall, we have to try to eat more fresh foods that come from the ground and less stuff that comes from cans, boxes, bags and packages."*
> — "Human Lab Rats" ELYGAD

We tend to spend lots of our hours of our days indoors. When we do get out it is too often just from the door to the car. We drive to our destination and keep our shoes clean walking mainly on the pavement. That has become a normal part of our lifestyle. As a result, we are losing some of our human instincts. We used to know how to heal ourselves with our minds. But we lost our ability to hear our internal voices. We can hear the jingles of the tell-lie-vision ads calling us instead of our innate inner guides.

As natural beings, our connection with nature is absolutely essential to our survival. Some of the ways to re-connect include: meditating, fasting, camping, gardening, eating more live foods, sipping real fruit smoothies and pure herbal teas. We are meant to sustain ourselves with things fresh from the earth, things that are still alive and vibrating with the power of nature like we are. As adults we can still breast-feed from our Mother Earth, like newborns getting their "mother's milk". The very purpose of food is to nourish us and help us grow.

This modern day food is not only killing us, it is literally ruining our environment as well. Man, I remember how much I loved catching bees in jars and making them fight spiders with my boy Tony Clark when I was little. Seems like I rarely see those big, bumblebees anymore. Also almost every time it used to rain hard there would be dozens of worms up and down the sidewalks back in the day too. No more. On our road trips back then my dad had to use the window washer thing at the gas station to clean all the bugs splattered on the windshield. I go on road trips often and it seems to not be nearly as many bugs anymore. What is going on?

The weather is completely changing and natural disasters are occurring more sporadically – or is that just Haarp helping to manipulate it? Maybe both, but either way we can see clear indications that we are in danger of ruining our planet!

This is the result of all this genetically modifying movement that has taken place in America through corporations like Monsanto. This is why I urge you to take your support away from huge corporations. They are on the wrong team. In America all the collusion, the chemtrails, the factory farms and the blatant abuse of animals, land, people and insects in the name of commerce will yield an ugly karma from the earth.

I mean damn, there really aren't nearly as many bugs today! That is scary. I'm thinking if the bugs can't survive in this environment, exactly what makes us think we can?

If things like that don't wake us up and make us realize we need to changes, I don't know what will.

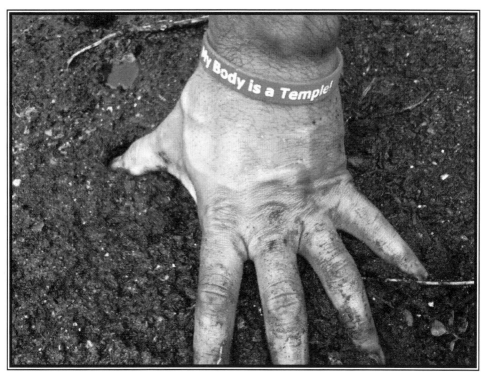

When is the last time you ran your bare hands through the soil? We should periodically take off our shoes and socks and walk barefoot in the soil. That is how we can reconnect with our essence anytime.

HOW AMAZING IS MOTHER EARTH?

> *"...in the abundance of water, the fool is thirsty..."*
>
> *Rat Race* ~ Bob Marley

One fall afternoon in Detroit I bumped into one of my old downtown Detroit neighbors Kim, who by that time was all but finished transforming into an awesome herbalist. Although I hadn't known her too well, I did recall her having a more regular, '9 to 5' type of job when we lived in the same building. I was a firefighter at that time. We laughed at the irony of how we both totally changed paths and became light workers. She was glowingly excited to know that she had found her true path and purpose in life – I know that feeling all too well. There is so much joy that comes along with self-discovery.

She was sharing some of the amazing things she'd learned about the world of herbs, healing and life in general. She explained how right in our own yards, herbs sprout up based on the needs of our bodies! They will grow right there around us, for us, in direct response to what we need to heal and balance ourselves. That is how in tune nature is with us – as we neglect and don't know how to utilize Mother Nature.

In our ignorance, we tie up our shoes and walk down the sidewalk paying no attention to the many wild herbs we pass. We mow a lot of them down every week or perhaps even spray killer chemicals on them! We head to pharmacies or doctors' offices to spend big money on some man made chemical imitations of the herbs similar to the ones we zoom right pass. Looking for the chemist in a white coat to cure us. When actually our healing can be found within our beings and right within the nature that surrounds us. She explained how the land where we spend that much time is connected with us in a sense, so much that right in our own yard the herbs that will help heal us will just pop up.

The whole idea of that connection is completely fascinating to me! The earth where we dwell can connect with us, but today we fail to take enough time out to connect with Mother earth. That is a relationship that we definitely need to actively forge. This is why it is good to get out and be barefoot in the soil. We have become products of our environment. How sad is it that we know the schedule of all of our favorite television programs, but have no idea what phase or sign the magnificent moon is currently in. In my eyes it seems like that is really ignoring God in a way. Those are natural guides that are there for a purpose. That is another glaring example of our modern day disconnection with nature.

It is important that we keep up with the elements of nature. We have to proactively do things that will keep us balanced – like having our plants, stones and crystals present in our homes/apartments. Even hugging and speaking to some of the trees we walk pass. Turn the cell phone off, leave it at home and get out to the park to walk or meditate in nature for an hour when you can – breathe in that fresh air and connect with nature. These things are important in order for us to stay grounded in the digital world. Take advantage of the natural resources that are available.

We are all surrounded by nature. My talk with Kim about herbs reminded years back when I'd first meant with **Dr. Isis** in Detroit. She really helped to open me up to new levels of overstanding and ever important self-acceptance. I had seen her health flyers for years and wondered who was doing that in the hood. She makes her own ads – 21 steps towards a healthier lifestyle and things like that – they would be posted right on top of the sleazy malt liquor posters in the grimiest party stores around Detroit. I always thought that was so revolutionary, it's always inspired me.

Dr. Isis and I were talking one random beautiful summer afternoon the universe had us cross paths in Detroit. We were talking as we rode our bikes through an average, run down neighborhood. She told me to get of the bike and walk with her for a minute; she wanted to show me something. We walked and she pointed around vacant houses and lots, in various yards, on the side of the freeway and even down the litter filled, pee-wreaking alleys – she was pointing at what I would have called tall weeds. "You see that over there, that is such and such root...the yellow is this...the purple over there, that is such and such."

I was flabbergasted. She explained how she would easily gather and work with many different types of wild herbs found right around the city. Wow! Products of our environment indeed, nature is giving us medicine. The best things in life are indeed free but our minds also have to be free enough to accept and attract that type of knowledge. We have to learn to work with the tools that nature continuously provides for us. I look at the side of the freeway in Detroit sometimes and think how we are rolling right pass a colorful and free herb garden. Literally.

I have read how dogs instinctively know how to medicate themselves with various herbs, when we assume they are eating grass they are actually soothing themselves with various wild herbs. They follow their natural instincts; we trust doctors and drug companies. Perhaps we should be learning from them in that case. We should always be in some form of communication and feel a connection with the trees, the moon, the stars and our angels.

Still buzzing from the awesomeness of nature I was sharing the connectivity story with my people **Roxanne Moore**, another of the many light workers in my circle. She is very well versed in the area of herbs and has started our own herbal-based company **Love Earth Herbal.**

Not only was she not surprised at all by the connectivity of earthly herbs to our needs – she also added more to it. She shared with me that she heard that in areas where a lot of cigarette smokers are found, the wild herb Mullein inevitably grows. Mullein has a long history of being good for many things, especially coughs and lung issues. Wow. So smokers cough and nature responds? Damn…that's incredible.

Nature tries her best to look out for us, but we simply ignore so many of her gifts. For instance, I remember how nobody liked having Dandelions in their yard. Back in the day my mom having me fertilize the grass as soon as it gets warm in attempts to get the jump on and defeat the dreaded Dandelions year after year. They even used to break through the tiny cracks of the cement – had to spray stuff on them or use a butter knife to dig them out. Now as an adult I am reading this online:

> Dandelion is a great spring tonic for our bodies; it helps the transition from winter to the warmer season, by nourishing and balancing the blood so it will flow better and keep us cooler in the summer season.

What?! It goes on to list many health benefits and great things about the dandelion root. Noting that it contains lots of zinc, iron and potassium.

We are talking about that same resilient "weed" that frustrated my mom so when they multiplied in our yard. She had us hand picking them with a spoon, making sure to dig up the root to ensure they wont return. That same dandelion is actually a really healthy herb? I was shocked to see the long list of good things that it does. Both the leaves and roots of dandelion can be used in numerous ways. Who knew? Something that is very healthy is readily available to us all, for absolutely free? And it pops up in the springtime just when our body needs it? Well damn. That just shows me we just have to be more tuned in; nature is teaching us how to prep our bodies for the cycles of nature!

This all reiterates what I was saying in ELYGAD, we have to stop thinking of living healthy as being too expensive. That is the easy copout. Living naturally has much less to do with money than it does to do with investing time learning the resources that are abundantly available and how to utilize them. We have to spend is more time learning more about our amazing Mother Earth. Make that investment.

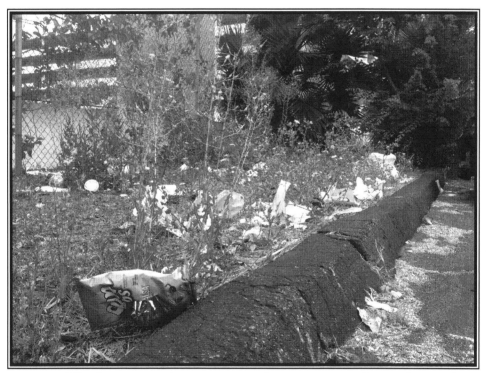

Even in middle of concrete jungles our awesome planet wants to supply us with many things that we can use for FREE! How do we thank her? Ignore it walk right past it on the way to the pharmacy. We'll even casually dump our trash and wrappers in fields full of medicine.

CREATE YOURSELF A SAFE PLACE

There is no place like home. The outside environment is quite polluted. We really want to keep the unnatural energy of the outside world OUT of our homes. In essence, making our own personal space a safe places at the crib.

Everyone knows the environmental challenges that we face in this modern world. We hear about all the things that "they" do: they put more and more artificial ingredients inside our foods and beverages. They experiment on us with genetically modified foods, which they refuse to even put a label on in the U.S. New medicines are approved without lengthy or proper testing. **Our EPA, FDA and USDA are all on the same BS.** They put fluoride into our municipal water supplies. 4G and Wifi signals fill up the air and our bodies as everyone surfs away on our smart phones. We look up and can watch as 'they' play tic tac toe in the skies with chemtrails.

Some things are literally out of our reach and control.

However, we can control our own nest and temple. Since we can't control the air outside of our living space—**we should assume some control and work to *limit* the amount of toxins that our families are exposed to inside of our homes.** Our homes should be a safe place.

It's like we discussed in *Eat Like You Give a Damn*, how we cannot control the food industry but we can work to limit the amount of processed foods we allow into our own bodies. The same principal applies here.

The fact that we cannot control something does not mean that we should lay down and play into the corporation's hands. We have to create alternatives and grasp control of all that we can. Some simple adjustments can help us assume control of the energy of our homes.

Keeping our households balanced with humanity, hand crafted things, book, plants, art, music, gemstones/crystals, laughter and love is in itself a powerful protective barrier from the capitalistic society that surrounds us. Those are very important elements to a safe and natural home.

We have to learn to produce more goods, food and medicines made in our very own loving energy, filling our homes with our own products.

Balance human energy with the digital world inside your home. **Kill that TV and log off some nights to tune into the high definition of the stars and the moon.** Connect with nature and utilize the natural power that we all possess. Close your eyes and meditate a shield of peace, love and harmony around your room, apartment or home.

Burn sage periodically to cleanse the air and energy in the house. Use that as your air freshener instead of the leading brand aerosol spray. Keep some in the bathroom.

Consider creating a small alter or place where you can quietly meditate inside the house. Place pictures of your ancestors and symbols of things you aspire to in that area. Designate your own convenient and private place to escape for peaceful moments where you can block out the problems of the outside world. You can have your morning or evening tea there with your ancestors and angels. Visualize and create the things you want for the upcoming days. Meditation is a powerful tool that makes anything possible.

These are the types of things that help make our homes safe places that give us peace and love that we can always have with us.

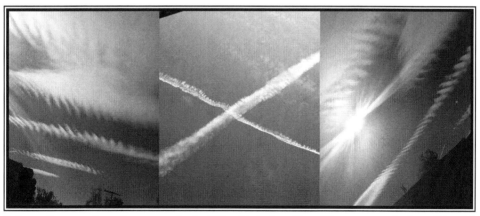

Exhaust from airplanes have never looked like this before. Ever. These strange looking "clouds" constantly fill our skies too often. And did you see people all over the country taking fire to that fake "snow" that didn't melt and turned black? It looked like Styrofoam or something. WTH is up with that? It's just unbelievable what these fools will do to manipulate our environment. I hope now you see more clearly what I mean by the artificial world.

EASY-TO-GROW PLANTS THAT CAN
HELP CLEAN THE AIR OF YOUR HOME

One way to proactively create a safe place in your home is getting one of these air-purifying houseplants.

Plants already bring new energy and life into your living space. Understanding that we can also use them for important purposes – like purifying our air – indicates just how much we can benefit from simply working with nature. So many of the things that we need can be provided affordably by nature. We have to see the value in that.

Part of the message of this book is that we value the wrong things in this society. It's funny that there is such a popular belief that it takes loads of money to lead a healthy lifestyle today – when all it may really take is a reconnection with nature. We have to realign our own priorities and learn to invest in natural things.

Making one of these easy to grow houseplants a member of our family is an excellent starting point. Have fun with it. Give them a name and talk to them – offer love and attention along with fresh water (if you give them tap water, let it sit outside for 30 minutes first). Explain their purpose to them of helping to make the air healthy for your family and thank them for doing so.

In return they will give us love back and work hard to help rid our homes of harmful toxins, and even odors like cigarette smoke – cleaning the air around the clock. Plus they will be adding lots of beauty and life to our living spaces.

Introducing some of these beautiful and affordable plants in our homes equates to instantly adding an advanced air quality control team to your home – for just a few bucks. It is certainly worth it for our family.

It could help make the home more comfortable for those with allergy and asthma type symptoms. Adding a plant or two to help keep the air of our home clean is definitely seems like a low risk, high reward step towards overall health.

Most of these are plants that you have seen before…
<u>**THE PLANTS:**</u>
1) Spider Plant

This elegant plant is great at removing poisonous gases as well as other impurities like formaldehyde and xylene. Try one near your kitchen.

2) Aloe Vera

We know that aloe vera can be used in many skin care products. Not only does it help with skin but it also with filtering various gas emissions from dangerously toxic materials. Aloe possess tons of medicinal properties, this incredible plant can also be grown as an ornamental plant.

3) Chinese Evergreen (Aglaonema modestum)

Chinese Evergreen is a perennial plant that is an excellent air-purifying plant. A very common houseplant that is really easy to grow – it thrives even better with less water and minimum light. It can also filter out airborne toxins such as benzene and formaldehyde. Good one to have.

4) Snake Plant

Snake Plant is one that is very popular and very easy to grow. It is a perennial that can also make it with less or even irregular water and light. But it these plants can serve an important purpose, Scientists at NASA have found out that this plant has the amazing ability to absorb formaldehyde, nitrogen oxides, and a variety of other chemicals present in the air. Not a bad idea to have one around our homes.

5) Peace Lily

Peace Lily is known to reduce harmful indoor toxins that may cause cancer. An easy-to-care-for houseplant, the peace lily is a strong pollution fighter and air-purifier. It helps in removing benzene and formaldehyde present in the house.

6) Rubber Plant

The Rubber Plant is tough and can tolerate dim or cooler living conditions, making it a great choice for a houseplant. They are easy to grow and great for removing chemical toxins from the house, particularly formaldehyde. The leaves of a rubber plant however can be poisonous for dog, keep that in mind.

Here are some other notable plants that have been proven to improve the air quality of the home:
- Gerber daisy
- Golden pothos
- Warneck dracaena
- Chrysanthemum
- Red-edged dracaena
- Bamboo palm
- Weeping fig
- Azalea
- English Ivy

MOOD ENHANCEMENT
Studies have also shown that plants can naturally help to improve your mood. Keeping some of these beautiful elements of nature close will not only cleanse the air, it can help bring a smile on your face as well. ☺

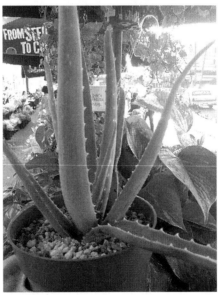

The amazing Aloe Vera plant has many, many potential uses.

ALOE VERA

One of the major focuses of this book is finding ways to replace the commercial products at the local pHARMacies with more natural products.

The Aloe plant is a perfect example of just how much we can do with awesome nature. Aloe not only helps to keep the air of our home clean, but it has many other useful functions as well:

- **Sun/Razor/Cooking Burn Products** – After losing a bout with the hot South Beach sun, many people go to the drugstore for a sunburn relief product of some sort. They are usually Aloe based, but of course they have some industrial ingredients added. We could just as easily break off a piece of our Aloe plant and rub the gel right into our skin for razor, sun or kitchen burns. It is cooling and 100% natural. Best of all it costs virtually nothing. And the plant will keep growing.

- **Hair Products** – Aloe gel helps to relieve the conditions of **dermatitis seborrheic** and **Psoriasis**. It can be used for hair products in a variety of ways. Aloe is a staple ingredient in most commercial hair conditioners. It is good for **dry hair**, and I've used it to **twist my locs** – it works perfectly for that too. All my D-I-Yers out there, it's a good base for your custom hair care products.

- **Face Astringent/Acne products** – Aloe gel can be used as a face astringent that will gently and naturally cleanse deep into the face.

- **Massage Oils/Products** – On a hot day take a gooey cool gel of Aloe and tell your significant other to lay down for a refreshing back rub with it. It is the perfect slippery, slimy texture – and good for the skin. It can be used as a **personal lubricant** as well – it is condom safe and pH balanced as well.

- **Wound Healing Products** – Aloe has been shown to help assist the body in healing wounds. Treat your scars with aloe and vitamin E and watch them vanish.

Investing in a large Aloe plant will pay big dividends because it can be used for so many different things. **It seems we will all be richer once we understand that we can find all that we need to maintain ourselves in nature.**

COMPOSTING
(Recycling Food)

Mom always reminded us that there are children starving in this world as she told us not to waste our food. She was right. It's not cool at all to waste food in a society with hungry people. To take it a step further **composting** is something that we should all seriously consider making a normal practice in our households. That is another way to make sure we aren't being wasteful.

While mom is cooking, instead of wasting stems, seeds, peels and scraps of foods by throwing it in the trash or down the disposal – collecting it for compost is a way to utilize it all. That way it will ultimately become part of the soil that will feed new plants, allowing all parts of the plant to serve a purpose in the circle of life. How appropriate?

After writing/reading this, I think all the time how wasteful to keep tossing out the middle part of a green pepper or all of those stalks of the broccoli. It is quite irresponsible in a way. So many seeds are just wasted when cut and use peppers.

Composting is a fairly easy thing to start implementing at home. The house would then be producing less garbage in general. We should become much more familiar with the idea of both separating and minimizing our waste; those are still relatively new concepts in America. In order to preserve our beautiful planet we have to begin to think and operate more mindfully.

It could be as simple as getting a large Tupperware container to store in the freezer and on a daily basis collecting compostable food scraps in it. We can easily find a family member, local gardener or a community garden to drop it off at periodically.

A **compost bin** or a **composting starter kit** for the house is another idea very much worth exploring. Check it out next time you are online. There are several different kinds on the market for indoor and outdoor use. Compost bins are airtight so there is no odors or worry of fruit flies.

A **Vermicomposting kit** (complete with worms), actually gives us a way to create our own dynamic soil to grow our own plants, herbs and food in. I love that. Make your own dirt. We can all love the fact that we are being green and not wasting food. It's a win-win.

Vermicomposting is the process of worms, usually red wigglers, breaking down kitchen scraps into nutrient rich organic matter. It makes some of the absolute best fertilizer in the world. It's a perfect little project for children in classrooms and families as well. The kids can feed and care for the pet worms and the parents use the finished product for the garden.

With the current dangers of our modern food industry looking like they will continue to worsen, **take this time to emphasize the importance working with nature to our future generations.** Making composting a regular thing in our households is a perfect way to set that ball in motion.

For more information on vermicomposting check out the book *Worms Eat My Garbage* by Mary Appelhof.

THE CIRCLE OF LIFE

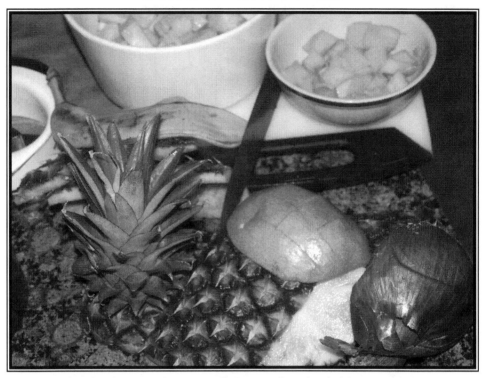

In the health food stores there are all types of seed oils like Lemon, Apricot or Grapefruit seed oil. The skins and roots can be used in a lot of different ways as well. It should make us realize that all of the parts of a plant are important. Just think how each little seed could potentially grow into a massive fruit-bearing tree itself. There is a lot of potential in those seeds; and the skins are often the most nutrient dense part. We should definitely utilize all that energy for something.

So much of the brilliance of nature is casually wasted as we toss the seeds and stems into the trashcan. Composting allows us to reinvest that energy back into the earth.

Both gardening and composting are things that could help bring us back to our own human roots. Indigenous people of this land were well known to have a profound respect for land, nature and animals. Today we have gotten too far away from that and need to inch back in that direction. This is a great way to start.

THE SHRINKING BOOKSHELF

When I was little we came home from a family vacation to find that someone had broken in the house and stolen our damn Encyclopedias. It was awful. I remember the Detroit police coming and pretending to do the fingerprint thing and all that. The thief apparently couldn't carry them all, but volumes like A – K were gone! The naked shelf looked so odd after being so used to seeing it filled with big books.

It's so interesting to me looking back that a set of books was easily one of the most valuable items that we had in the house. Even the petty thief, who is probably not the most avid reader in the world, knew that. Things are much different now.

As technology booms it is an unfortunate fact today that the value of books is decreasing. As a writer and publisher this is certainly something I am very aware of. I still love the feel of holding books. I personally haven't gotten into the whole e-book thing just yet although it is probably inevitable. I really enjoy the process of signing and dating my books for people. I put so much thought and energy into creating it, in my eyes it is my version of a work of art. Picasso baby. But then again…so is an iPad.

With the recent boom of electronic reading devices, the Internet, smartphones, social networks and bloggers – the actual physical book market is swiftly decreasing. I encourage you to keep collecting books and value your book collection! It can mean a lot, especially for young people to have that access to knowledge right inside the house. Remember that all of this electronic stuff can crash, malfunction or not power up at anytime. Take pride in those bookshelves because knowledge is the real power.

vs.

THE GROWING REFRIGERATOR

On the other hand, one thing that is certainly not going anywhere in food-brained America is the refrigerator. They are huge. Of course where else would we keep leftovers and store tomorrow and the next day's catch of the day? And just in case the massive double door fridge doesn't have enough room for everything, sometimes we keep another big ass freezer down in the basement too!

When I talk to my friends from other countries around the world, they always seem to make note of how large the refrigerators are here in America. Fridges aren't as big in any other country. They are not as accustomed to the idea of storing large amounts of food – that is just a habit that we have adopted over here in the good ole land of the fat, I meant free.

When my first version of ELYGAD was finally done I wanted all of my friends to have it immediately! I was literally giving it away left and right. It didn't seem as important to my people as I thought it should. I eventually came to the realization that it wasn't just me or my book that wasn't particularly intriguing to them – the fact was a lot of people around me didn't really buy and read books all that often. In 2009 it is estimated that 'black' Americans dropped 7.4 billion dollars on hair/personal care, 18.6 billion in phone services but only 31 million on books. We do not value books as much as we should.

That's how I came up with the idea of the refrigerator versus the bookshelf! I want to remind young people to keep a book collection and have us all do some self-evaluating.

In my perfect world, I insist that every home in America should have at *least* enough books to match the capacity of your refrigerator(s). I thought that was a pretty fair balance on the minimum end. That can certainly say a lot about one's priorities. But hell, you never know, the way they keep people under educated and extra food brained in America, they might as well change the slogan to '*eating* is fundamental'. #IJS

> "*...before I date a man, I need to see what his bookshelf is looking like...*"
> —Jessica Care Moore

I hear that! Now that's some real game.

SIMPLE FENG SHUI

Feng Shui is another tool to help control the energy and flow of energy in our homes. This is an ancient Chinese practice that originates in Chinese astronomy. It is a very deep science; In order to simplify and easily begin to apply it in the western world we can use what is called the Bagua of the 8 Aspirations. The Bagua map is used to map a room or building and see how the different (directions) sections correspond to different aspects in our lives.

The basic Bagua Grid looks like this:

Wealth	Reputation & Fame	Relationships & Marriage
Family Ancestors & Inspiration	Health & Well-being	Children
Knowledge & Self-cultivation	Career	Travel & Helpful people

Align this side with the main entrance of your home, room or office.

We could even use this system of Feng Shui on the surface of our desk in our workspace. How else could we apply this in our lives? We could take advantage of the grid and place some pictures of places we want to travel in the 'travel corner' of the home. In the wealth corner we can place a large plant that will continue to grow and symbolize our own growing abundance. This is a way to approach all of the different directions, put symbols of things that we aspire. Consider it like an interactive vision board with some added dimensions.

It is ridiculously expensive for a small publisher to print books in full color, but there are also colors that correspond with each cardinal direction or section of the grid. Make sure to look up the 'Bagua grid' online. Place gemstones and crystals in the appropriate places, program them and put them to work for you. For instance, explain the exact type of relationship that you wish for in detail to a beautiful Rose Quartz crystal – then place it in the Relationship corner. We can attract exactly the things we desire by using more of the resources that are available to us.

Products of Our Environment

The Mercury Retrograde (pg 124) period is a great time to **rede**corate and **re**organize. Take advantage of that time and do some evaluation. Shift some things around to attract new energy into specific areas of our lives where it is needed. That's a perfect way to start getting your Feng Shui on! These age-old practices like this one are still around for a reason.

You will find that one of the main focuses in this book is that we all begin to acknowledge and educate ourselves on natural tools like Feng Shui, astrology, numerology, reflexology, yoga, meditation, tantra, tarot cards, chakras, stones and crystals. **These things are virtually free products of our environment** that can help us to get in sync with the energy flow of our universe. Those things can be utilized to align ourselves with the forces of nature puts them to work for us. And there is no limit to how high we can soar with Mother Nature's wind at our backs.

Once we find and work towards our purpose in life we can easily harness the power of the universe around us. Use the tools to create a life that is a fantastic voyage.

STONES AND CRYSTALS

Do yourself a favor and **take a slow stroll through a stone/crystal shop. It is a very peaceful experience. Feel your way around and pick up the ones that catch your eye.** Take a few minutes to fondle it while you are in the store. Explore your connection with different stones and learn about some of their purposes. You might discover something that you really needed. There are many different types of stones for every purpose, including aiding in healing different parts of the body, focus, communication, meditation, abundance, protection and much more.

Yes…we go spend big money on doctors and dangerous prescriptions with harmful side effects when something as natural as stones can help facilitate healing in our bodies. We don't take advantage of these really accessible products of our environment. We tend to opt for the man made ones.

How the stones/crystals "work" is by transferring energy – it is the power of nature. Everything is vibrating with energy and these stones are literally hundreds of thousands of years old. They carry an ancient energy and wisdom with them.

You can tap into that energy and actually program stones for specific purposes. Holding the stone tightly in your right hand, assign it a purpose and put it to work for you.

Remember each zodiac sign has several corresponding stones, that is a good way to get started in the stone/crystal world. Give someone you care about his or her birthstone along with the description.

We can use them in many practical ways. Students can carry and use a piece of **Flourite**, which is a wonderful stone to use for the absorption of information and knowledge. Study with it and put it on your desk during a big exam.

Citrine is a stone of good luck and creativity. It is known to promote success, prosperity and abundance. If you are experiencing writers or creative blocks for instance, citrine is the perfect way to remove it. This is a good stone to put in the wealth corner of your living space as it vibrates abundance!

The amazing **Black Tourmaline** is a most powerful protector. Like *all* **black** stones, it helps neutralize electromagnetic frequencies. **Black Tourmaline though has the awesome ability to actually repel negative vibrations and energies of all kinds** – keeping negativity away from us! Use them in your home or workplace around the computers and flat screens. Let your children keep one in their pockets or backpacks in order to keep them protected when they are out in the matrix.

Those are just some basic ways to utilize the energy of stones and crystals. Of course they are great for meditation and many other things. I highly encourage you to work with these awesome products of nature.

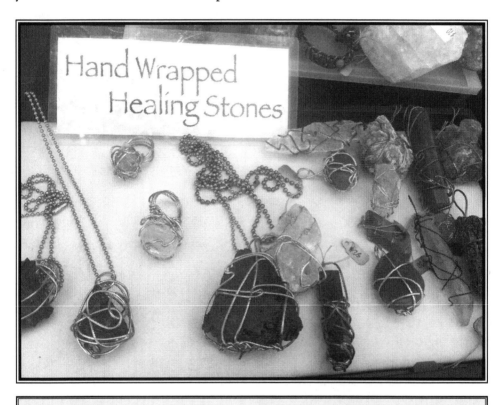

This section of the book gets tough for my old school Christian readers. They are often not open to things like this. Some might even think of it is as dark or devilish type of stuff. But it is even right in the Bible – in the book of Ezekiel chapter 28, it talks about the 12 stones/crystals used to make the Holy breastplate. In Revelations it mentions the 12 crystals that were used to make the wall of the New Jerusalem. So please don't foolishly ignore these awesome gifts of nature that come from the Creator. Nature is God. Become open to a new level of understanding.

Speaking of power, this an example of how amazing these gemstones/crystals are:

MOLDAVITE

Soon after I really dove into the world of stones and crystals I came across Moldavite. Moldavite is actually not a stone or crystal, its a Tektite, meaning it has a meteoric origin. It was the first stone that I felt a very strong vibration from instantly. As soon as I held it in my hands, I could feel light pulsing heat that continued to increase. I connected with it like the guy in Avatar did with that flying horse thingy. I read the corresponding card; I was in complete awe of what I was actually holding inside my hands!

Check this sh*t out:

> *Moldavite is the product of a meteor collision with the Earth nearly 15 million years ago. It fell over what is now called the Moldau River valley in the Czech Republic. These green gems are among the most rare minerals on earth. They have been prized by humans for thousands of years and are still given as gifts from royalty to royalty. In legend, it is believed Moldavite was the green stone in the Holy Grail and has the power to quicken one's spiritual evolution.*
>
> *Even people not normally sensitive to the energies of stones, often feel the energy of Moldavite. Many sense it as heat, tingling, or a pulsing sensation in their hand. Others feel a rush of energy through their body, usually upwards out the top of their head. Moldavite's high vibrational energy is a powerful chakra opener, particularly at the heart and above. Sleeping with Moldavite activates the Dreams State. Wearing it helps manifest positive life change.*

Yes, that says **15 MILLION** years ago! So wait, this is a little piece of an actual meteorite from millions of years ago? Wow! That's like the type of stuff that gives out super powers in the movies or some sh*t. But this is real life.

That is some heavy stuff. One thing that we should learn is energy NEVER dies! Holding something that old, that is still vibrating in my hand literally _millions_ of years later. Man! How could we not want to connect with something like that? Put that iPhone down for a minute and grab a hold of some of nature's amazing technology!

That is so much older than any of our 'his-story' books even taught us the world even is. Imagine the stories this thing must have. Meditate and talk with it! Put it under your pillow at night. Those stars that we gaze at on clear nights that we know are way far, far away in another galaxy – this is a little piece of one of them? That is way exciting! That is some real bling-bling.

That is the type of thing that we should keep around the house and on our person. It keeps us grounded in this digital world we exist in today. We should definitely take advantage of these mind-boggling acts of nature. It is unbelievable.

So here is yet another world of wonderful tools that nature has right at our disposal. All we have to do is understand that they exist and take advantage of them.

Damn…life is good. ☺

MAINTAINING BALANCE IN THIS MATRIX

Yes, it is very hard to completely avoid the corporate products that line the shelves of every store and gas station in America. What we have to do is strive to maintain some kind of balance.

As re-iterated many times in this book, try not to let all of the products you use and eat come from huge corporate energy. In order to make sure you are maintaining some balance, keep some of the elements of nature around.

Keep a couple gemstones/crystals in your home or office – or on your person. Wear gemstone jewelry on precious metals of gold, copper or silver. They are not only beautiful but also have a specific purpose.

Some of those stones are hundreds of thousands, even millions of years old! As living beings, we want to hold on to something like that. They contain the intricate magnificent power of earth and nature inside them – along with the wisdom of our ancestry. Take advantage of these very affordable and all-powerful resources.

Essential oils provide the same kind of dual functionality. Not only do they smell great, they also have various medicinal, protective and anti-bacterial properties. Build a collection of oils that can be used as our cologne/perfume and in air fresheners – plus be used in many homemade cosmetics and medicines.

Have some plants around your home. Surround yourself with things that remind you to appreciate nature and natural processes. Plants can help clean the air and add color and life into your space.

Hang original **artwork** around your home to add color and bring vibrancy to your living area. Value those old school, **hand crafted antiques** for their human element and the simple beauty of our creations.

Make it a point to be more aware and align your habits with the cycles and movements of the moon and stars. Begin your new projects with the new moon and let them grow with the waxing moon. Cleanse your stones/crystals under the full moon. Get rid of unwanted habits during the waning moon.

Bake things from scratch at home instead of buying packaged cookies and snacks. Lick the batter off the spoon. Enjoy the unique and not so perfectly round shape of each one. Let that unforgettable smell fill your house. Remember to enjoy and respect the entire process.

We have to conserve old-fashioned ways that will enable us to maintain our balance in this corporate world.

Most people now begin realizing that they live in the matrix. What most people don't realize is that the matrix lives in them.

> *Whenever we permit sodas, candy bars, junk food, and cigarettes to enter our body, we're letting the energies and vibes of corporations, factories, offices, CEOs, and executives into our very being. These are the active ingredients of the matrix.* — Alok

ANTI CORPORATION
Be You-nique

I still love to take my plain tee shirts, cut off the sleeves and write Anti-Corporation or one of my other slogans neatly across the chest. Sometimes I don't want to rock any name brand. Even in that small capacity I like feeling the freedom that accompanies self-expression. I personally like to see people tatted up and creatively dressed – expressing their own unique styles and swag. Though we are all connected, we all have our own forms of self-expression. We should always honor that. I would not be surprised at all to find myself morphing into a mid-life, tatted up temple.

When I say anti-corporation, I mean it on many levels. One aspect of it is that we should not spend our invaluable life energy or creativity working for the gain of corporations that only care about money. Too often we are supporting conglomerates that exploit impoverished areas and are not earth friendly in their practices. They want to keep us in the dark about what they feed our families.

We are all born artists, farmers, musicians, healers, teachers, dancers, athletes, **vegetarians**, engineers and architects – not line workers. God didn't create line workers. Corporations did.

We have to find ways to use our energy to work for humanity in some capacity. Don't work a job that you don't even like. We are all born with an innate and unique gift/purpose to offer this universe. Share it with us! Use your gift to do something that will help make our world a better place.

We have to discover and identify what our true gifts are and then build a career and life around those things. That is our duty. Get your zodiac chart done and pay close attention to what out what is in your 2nd house (resources), 6th house (daily duties), and 10th houses (career). Those are the money and work houses of your chart. That can provide some tremendous insight into the type of work that you should pursue.

Once we begin to break free and move in that direction, the universe will gladly assist us down that path. Working with the tools of nature (astrology, numerology, gemstones/crystals), can help us find our gifts and discover our path.

That is one of the aspects of Anti-Corporation. Another one that has been continuous throughout this book is cutting our support of huge corporations through commercial products. It is well documented that many of these companies have ultimately placed financial gain over the common good of humanity. Many of them also support this Genetically Modified madness, which is not something that we want to help fund at all. We can't even get them to at least label the damn GMO's finally in America. How horrifying is that – what they feed us is a mystery? Crazy!!!

Why Do They Want to Keep Our Ingredients Secret?

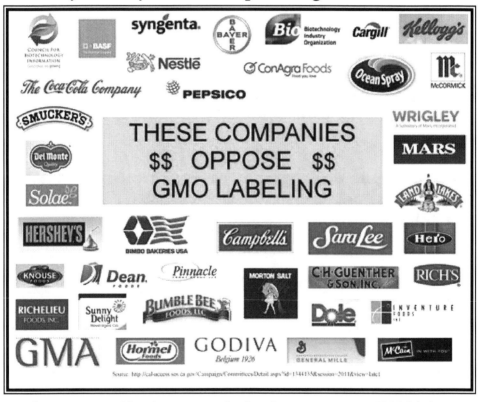

These companies (above) came up with a lot of money to oppose GMO labeling.

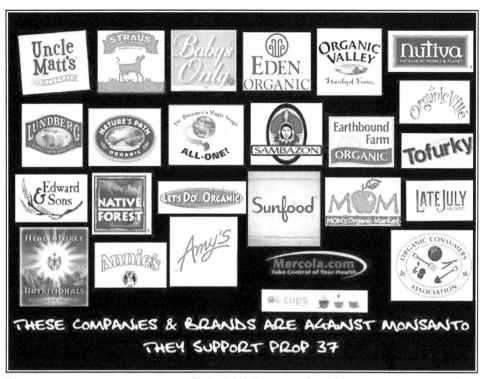

THESE COMPANIES & BRANDS ARE AGAINST MONSANTO THEY SUPPORT PROP 37

These companies were in support of GMO labeling. We should limit our support to those who support us.

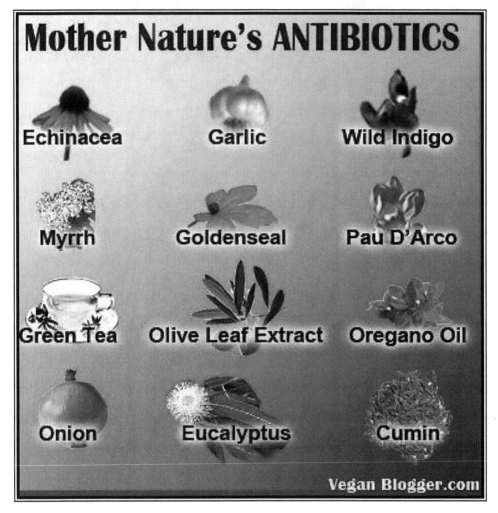

Health and healing has to begin inside of the home. Running to the doctor or the local drug store has to become the **old** way of doing things.

The new way is to return to the ancient ways of mom being a healer and creating our own medicines and elixirs. We have to learn to harness our power as beings and work with nature.

When our children get a little cold, we don't have to run out to get a bottle of the leading brand cold medicine. Let that be the very last resort and not the first thought. First think about making your own loving cough syrup. Give them some warm Echinacea tea with lemon, and rub eucalyptus oil on their hands and feet. Wrap your own arms and healing energies around our loved ones is the way we begin caring for our families. Make fresh squeezed juices in your personal healing laboratory (kitchen).

Here are some natural antibiotic weapons that we can use to bring healthcare back into our own hands. Using these and other kinds of natural tools along with our own healing energy – there is nothing that our bodies are not capable of overcoming.

Fasting and **drinking lots of water** are two more inexpensive and effective preventative and healing medicinal ideas.

Silver is one of the original antibiotics of the world.

Antibiotics are fed to farm animals regularly in order to make them grow larger and to keep them alive in the filthy conditions of CAFO's. Nearly 80% of the total antibiotics sold in the US are used for farm animals. That practice is now leading to human resistance to the drugs.

These days, making sure we aren't eating meat from factory farming operations is a method of health insurance itself. I tell people that insist on eating meat all the time to find a family farmer in your area! It is just a simple google search away and then you have a meat man you can trust. Finding and dealing with a chicken farmer, a beef farmer or a fisherman is not at all hard. With the crazy conditions of commercial factory farming – it is definitely worth looking into.

It is time for use to be proactive in ensuring the health of our families. We know that it take a few extra steps today in order to do that.

Let's start taking them.

NATURAL HAIR GROWTH ENHANCERS

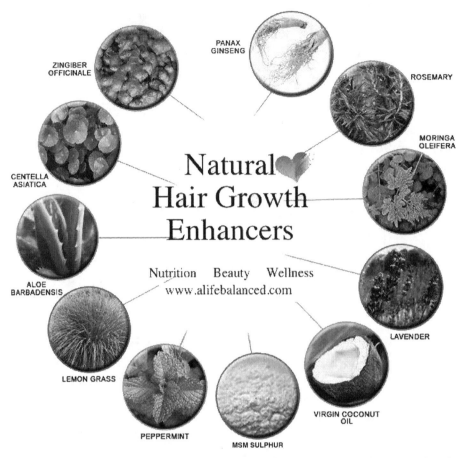

Natural ♥ Hair Growth Enhancers

Nutrition   Beauty   Wellness
www.alifebalanced.com

ZINGIBER OFFICINALE
PANAX GINSENG
ROSEMARY
MORINGA OLEIFERA
CENTELLA ASIATICA
ALOE BARBADENSIS
LAVENDER
LEMON GRASS
PEPPERMINT
MSM SULPHUR
VIRGIN COCONUT OIL

We are solution driven at Ra One Pubs. As we begin to adopt the idea of making our own products, here are some excellent potential building blocks. A lot of these ingredients we may commonly come across in trips to farmers markets or stores. It is time we think about collecting some of them and making our own healthy hair products!

With just a little creativity and patience, making our own custom body care products is very do-able. I want this book to open the door for a new way of thinking and inspire a generation of new producers.

Nothing can be better for us or hold the distinction of being custom made specifically for you, like making homemade products. Support local producers with hand made items. The human **love**, **energy** and **intention** will translate into unprecedented results. ☺

Products of Our Environment

This material points to many of the products that we use on a daily basis and exposes them as questionable – if not very dangerous. That subsequently creates a wide open market for those who want to create new options for us all. We need you right now.

We all deserve natural, healthy products made in good energy. In fact, we should begin expecting and demanding that quality. Our bodies are priceless; we only want the best for our temples! We should demand better quality from the brands that we support. Get online and voice your displeasure with them that way. Ask questions.

Of course everyone is not going to be interested in or have time to make his or her own products but by supporting those who do, instead of commercial producers, we will create a new generation of products that we can trust again.

Going forward we must stop running to the superstores for everything. Start wanting to know more about who is making your cosmetics and such. Take a quick look and learn a little more about what's inside that stuff.

Support quality items and goods that come from small, local companies that we can feel good about supporting, instead of huge corporations. Remember what your dollars are supporting on a larger scale. We want things hand made by people, not the dreaded products of mass production. Buying from a local source helps to rebuild and support the local economy, which ultimately strengthens the community.

AVOID PETROLEUM OR MINERAL OIL PRODUCTS

*(*Also known as **petrolatum**, **petroleum jelly** (Vaseline), **soft paraffin**, **white paraffin**, or even **mineral oil**.)*

> "...the shine in lip-gloss comes from petroleum jelly. Petroleum jelly is a byproduct of oil drilling, and when you spread it on your lips, you end up eating it, which is essentially the same as drinking gasoline. Add up the amount of lip-gloss the average woman uses (and consumes) over a decade, and it equals 7 pounds. The European Union has banned many petroleum jelly products, and experts are concerned they could be linked to cancer. Women with breast cancer have twice the levels of hydrocarbons (substances found in petroleum jelly) in their breasts than women who haven't had cancer...Steer clear of any products that list petroleum jelly or mineral oil on the ingredient list."
>
> —Dr. Oz

When I was growing up everyone had that big tub of Petroleum Jelly at the house. That is what we used for our lips, hair, skin and more. I wish I had known better. That is the way it is in my circle with Shea butter now. How I wish I had known about Shea Butter back then! I used to like to use 'baby' oil, which is mineral oil – meaning I was rubbing a liquid crude oil extract on my body temple? Damn. I simply had no idea what that stuff actually was. It was just what everybody used, nobody really talked about what it was.

I also used to cake that thick ass gasoline pomade in my hair and brush it with my Diane brush till my arms were sore trying to get 360 waves. The crazy things that go on daily that we don't know any better and do routinely are just baffling. Staggering. It is time we wake up! I could never imagine using that type of crap now under any circumstances. Impossible. There are just too many natural options that exist.

Petroleum, as in gasoline (!!), is a by-product of the distillation process in the production of fuel. It is cheap industrial waste material. It should not be used on our bodies at all. So many commercial products use **Petrolatum/Mineral Oil** in some form because it is so inexpensive. It is in basically **_all_** of the commercial cosmetics at large markets and drugstores. Every single one! Even some of the products found in health food stores still contain some form of Petroleum byproduct. Inspect those labels. Avoid that sh*t.

While people may be under the impression that petroleum/mineral oil based products provide moisture – that is not the case. It actually coats and clogs the pores of our skin, preventing it from breathing. It will effectively seal in moisture that is already present, but it also seals in toxins and prevents the body from breathing through the skin as it normally would. It suffocates the skin. Petroleum Jelly can even seal in the heat from a burn and make it worse.

I beg you not to put this shit on your babies! Don't feel bad if you didn't know and have been using petroleum-based stuff currently as you read this. That's ok. I used to use it too. All day. But now that you know what it is, you have to stop! Get rid of that crap. Start over simply with a good jar of Coconut Oil or Shea Butter. In the back of this book there is also a good list of completely natural brands.

Talk to your friends and family about this dangerous stuff too. I want your loved ones to be healthy and safe. I give you this information along with the responsibility of passing it on.

Yes ladies, they do have healthy alternative brands of lip-glosses as well. I have some of those listed or you can check at the local health food market, at least give some of the alternatives a try. It's imperative that we start making more informed decisions.

As stated throughout this book, shopping at American commercial markets will make it virtually impossible to avoid these ridiculous ingredients. I encourage you to shop at more local, health minded markets or online, always check the ingredients. Be on the lookout out for *any* of those "petro" words. No bueno! Look in the **POE** recipe section and learn to make a safe and simple '*non-petroleum*' jelly in minutes.

Always remember that anything you put on your porous skin will enter the blood stream 4 times faster than when you ingest it through the mouth. If you put something on your skin you should be able to eat it too. You do not want petroleum/petrolatum/propylene glycol/mineral oil or anything like that becoming a part of your blood system! Hell no! There are so many different types of natural butter and oil options. **Coconut oil, Shea butter, cocoa butter** or super soft **mango butter** are some tremendous upgrades from Petroleum based products.

The bottom line is that clogging the skin or scalp with petroleum and feeding a gasoline byproduct into our blood is not going to suffice any longer. Please start looking for more safe and sane options going forward.

A FEW GOOD PRODUCTS

There are some very good natural supplements that I have been fortunate to learn about and add to my list of 'must-have' products. I **highly** recommend that we all keep at least a few weapons like these in our health arsenal. The modern day lifestyle can be very hard on our bodies and we definitely need our Temples to last for many years. It is in our best interest to make a little effort to keep our system strong.

Regular use of the supplements listed here can provide very high quality, plant based nutrition that can quickly and conveniently be incorporated into our lifestyle. Eating properly today on a daily basis can be quite challenging for anyone. Taking any combination of these natural things consistently is a great idea to supplement any diet. We can feel very good knowing that we are giving our bodies a little something extra to work with.

These days the key is to form good habits and take advantage of the inexpensive things that are beneficial to your health, like mandatory daily shots of **Apple Cider Vinegar** or warm **Lemon water** every morning. Use those things as really simple and inexpensive forms of preventative medicines for your body. If we consistently provide our bodies with tools to work with we can more easily combat the lower quality, over processed foods that we are surrounded by daily.

The products highlighted in this chapter are seriously good for damn near EVERYTHING! You want to be taking them regularly. They are very affordable as well, (at least at Dhealthstore they are). Stock up when they are on sale. They can help you and they cannot harm you. Overdose on them. In my opinion, these are 3 things that should be in every household. There are so many things I would want to recommend, but these are a great start.

Moringa

This is another one of nature's divine gifts that we should take advantage of. **Moringa** is an absolute miracle plant that contains over 90 nutrients! It has literally everything inside it – from **essential fatty acids, calcium, zinc, iron** plus a high amount of our beloved **protein** – and much more. It actually makes a perfect supplement for **everyone of all ages**, especially for my vegans and vegetarians.

The highly nutrient dense Moringa, (I can't make an official claim), but the leaf alone can replace any multi-vitamin or pre-natal type of pills that we may be using. It is packed with a full spectrum of nutrients. It makes a great lactation aid for breast-feeding women and it can be used as a prenatal pill. It helps to make breast milk super nutritious. Fellas it is good to help replenish the body after fluid lost in the sex act.

It is useful for a number of important things in the body like balancing blood sugar and it is rich in iron therefore good for anemic conditions. Ladies it helps replenish fluids lost during the menstrual cycle. Truly, there is just not enough that can be said about Moringa, its good for flat out everything. Make sure you choose a trusted source and get the real deal – it is available in tea, oils, extracts, pills and all kinds of forms.

I remember a long time ago someone was telling me all about how this Moringa was a miracle tree, (in Latin the name Moringa literally translates into 'the Miracle Tree'). At that time I guess I just wasn't open to it. She had a lot of literature on it and all that – but it just sounded like a fad type thing to me. Like Noni juice or something. The sales pitch was kind of pyramid-like pushy and I really just blew it off.

I hadn't yet learned not be skeptical of everything and realize that I could gain valuable knowledge from many sources. The universe was sending me these gifts and I just wasn't ready. If you aren't familiar with Moringa, I encourage you to get familiar. Right away.

MSM Sulpher

Methylsulphonalmethane Sulpher is another one that is an all around great substance to supplement our lives. Simply put, everything on the body that grows, MSM Sulpher helps it to grow – including the hair, skin and nails. MSM is great for sore muscles, sprains and old athletic injuries – aiding in the repair of joints, tendons, bones and ligaments. It is an absolute must have for the aging athlete like myself!

The list of good things is almost too much to mention, make sure to do your own research on it. Among many things, MSM is known to be good for the prostrate and male reproductive system in general. It has detoxification properties and helps rid the body of parasites. Just like the two previous things listed here, it does just a host of good things. Seriously! It would benefit you to make it part of your daily routine.

Morning Time Tips

Each day is a new beginning. You can decide to begin making healthier choices any given morning. It's a good idea to make the very first thing you put in your body something simple and good. Set a good tone for the day.

For a great morning jumpstart, try adding a pinch of sea salt with a tablespoon of apple cider vinegar to a glass of room temp water. It is great tonic for the body overall – especially the joints, nervous system and the brain. That is another very affordable healthy tool worth adding to your lifestyle – it will greatly benefit the body in the long run. Take advantage of these types of things.

Hot water with lemon or Oil Pulling are a couple of affordable ways to mildly detoxify the body daily. For people who might have a hard time paying for or sticking with more demanding detox programs, these are some very affordable and effective options. Try it 21 days in a row! When you do things consistently the body can recognize the pattern and will begin to work with you. Strive to consistently start your days off right.

Black Seed Oil/Extract

Black Seed Oil is another must have health weapon that will bolster our immune systems in many ways. It has super strong medicinal properties and can be used for literally ANY adverse health condition that we can think of. It can be used internally and externally and a very little bit last a long time.

Black Seed oil is useful for treatment of tumors and therefore great for treatment of any type of cancer. It is also effective for any and all respiratory conditions (asthma, bronchitis, pneumonia, etc.). It also helps rid the body of worms and parasites. It is known to be good for high blood pressure and cholesterol as well. Damn near everything! Just like Moringa, Black Seed Oil can be used safely by anyone of all ages.

Be forewarned, black seed oil has a very intense taste. But just ½ of a teaspoon daily is awesome. To offset that have a lemon or orange wedge ready that's all.

I remember my friend the "Black Seed Lady" at Eastern Market in Detroit. She had the cough drops, lotions and many products made from Black Seed Oil. I used to love those candies. It's best to just take ½ teaspoon straight every day, trust me when I tell you **it will ruin a smoothie**. Back in those days I didn't realize how important these kinds of weapons were to maintain overall health. I was skeptical then, and just at the very beginning of my personal health journey.

All of you out there learn from my mistakes. Find a good source and keep some highly quality supplements like these around. Incorporate them into your daily routine. Stay away from the pharmacies, doctors and hospitals as much as possible.

Being healthy is not about money, but you should value your body enough to invest in it. I know lots of people who really don't care for supplements or popping pills. The modern day American food is leaving the body lacking so many important nutrients. Living in this matrix I personally feel that we really need to supplement our diet in some areas. I suggest keeping some high quality herbs as part of your daily intake. Unless you are really keeping up with your juice/smoothie game and growing your own produce and the whole thing, it's kind of hard to know for sure what is good these days.

Essential fatty acids (Omega 3-6-9) are important for many body functions. Please understand that you do not need fish oil to get it! **Black Currant Seed** oil, **Hemp Seed oil, Evening Primrose oil** and **Moringa Seed** oil are all rich in **Omegas 3, 6,** and **9.** The wild herb **Purslane** could be growing right in your hood for absolutely free, it too is rich in Omega 3, 6 and 9. Note that **flax seed** is high in Omegas 3 and 6 only.

One last thing I would suggest is slowly stocking up on **Ionic** Minerals such as: **Zinc, Copper, Iron, Silver, Selenium, Germanium,** etc. Get a couple on paydays or load up when they go on ½ off sale at Dhealthstore. Slowly build your collection. They last a long time and provide high quality minerals that are likely missing from the modern day, industrialized soil.

Take your time on your health journey and keep gradually improving. Add one tool at a time. Feel free to contact us with any questions or direction, we will be glad to help. Remember once you make up your mind that you want to begin to transition, you have to be open to new things because the Universe will continue to send you tool after tool in order to assist you.

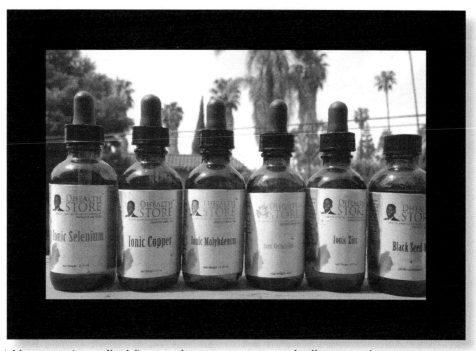

Adding ionic (not colloidal) minerals to your water periodically is a good way to compensate for the depleted American soil.

A FEW GOOD SOURCES

Sometimes people shop for vitamins at the local pharmacy or vitamin shop – maybe saving a few dollars. But that is definitely not the place to get our supplements from. We want should seek to get the finest quality herbs and vitamins we can, because that will be our medicine.

Remember that this book is all about knowing more about where our products are coming from and knowing the energy behind them. Look at the ingredients of some supplements from commercial sources we might notice extra ingredients and/or unnecessary fillers. I find it hard to trust that stuff. I try to avoid all commercial products in general, opting for higher quality products for my Body temple.

Be sure to check the bulletin boards of the local health food stores and yoga studios in our area for people offering local goods and services. If we seek those types of products we are sure to find them.

Herb N Life
herbnlife.myshopify.com

I love the name HerbNLife and can appreciate the quality of their product line. They offer a full line of body and hair care products that have completely natural ingredients – <u>nothing</u> beyond our understanding. Their Royal Rinse shampoo is one of my absolute favorites; it smells great and leaves a perfect royal tingle.

All of their products are high quality and they actually have "Love" listed as an ingredient. We all need to use products that are made with that loving energy. One day when my funds were lower, I checked out all of the less expensive brands at the health food store. All of them said pure and natural on the front of the labels – yet most of them had madness like **Petrolatum** and unnatural fragrance inside! No thank you! We are talking about our body temples, it is not enough to have 'mostly' good ingredients; I only deal with that all-natural quality. That's how I want you to roll from now on too.

Dehuty's Health Store
dhealthstore.com

It is so comforting to have a trusted and **affordable** source for getting natural products. After watching some of his videos and understanding what brother Dehuty Ma'at Ra and is all about, we will quickly see that this is the absolute perfect place to order our herbal supplements. I am done going to the health food store and overpaying for herbs.

Dhealthstore has the best variety of herbs. The ingredients are absolutely top quality and the customer service is first class – it has all of that going on and yet somehow **the prices are incredibly affordable!** Healthy stuff is always expensive right? I had gotten used to overpaying at the local health food stores, I don't even mind making that investment in my body temple. But then the universe led me to dhealthstore. I'll never overpay for vitamins/herbs again.

Dehuty Ma'at Ra is a master herbalist and life coach who keeps it way real. Anyone can see how much he truly loves what he does. I encourage everyone to support this store because they are absolutely doing things the right way and still keeping the prices below competitive. They carry a very wide and growing variety of natural products that will help us maintain a healthy lifestyle. We have to support businesses like this going forward. Start building a health arsenal at home with the quality products from **dhealthstore.com** right away.

BREATHE & S T R E C T H!

It is said that **the things that actually cause us to age are the loss of both water and flexibility in our bodies.** We have to remember to drink lots of water and keep our minds, limbs and organs lubricated and loose! We all get that wonderful morning wake up stretch to get days started. Don't forget we can enjoy that stretch throughout the day too.

It is refreshing to hear the sound of our children running and playing (at least when they used to actually go out and play instead of watching one of a 1,500 cable channels, playing video games or staring at each other's social network pages). In our modern day society, all of us, even the youth are becoming stiff and stagnant. As an adult, when was the last time that you ran absolutely as fast as you could? It has been quite a while for most of us. Our legs and hearts can use that exercise!

S t r e c h i n g can be a good reminder for us to slow down and consciously use our entire being to gradually expand on what our previous limits were. Our minds, muscles and breathing techniques all must patiently learn to work together. That alone makes it great exercise! Even if it is only 15 quiet, isolated minutes in the morning and the same in the evening, the daily practice of stretching can be very beneficial.

There is a good life metaphor involved with stretching our bodies. Being flexible and readily able to adjust and adapt will prove to be a very valuable life skill. In fact, I had the thought that **perhaps remembering to reach as far as you can everyday will actually help you reach as far as you can in your life.** In this vast world and universe, we should always expand our thoughts and seek to use our magnificent minds and bodies to their full potential! There is absolutely no limit to what we can do if we set our mind to it.

Too often the routine of life has us so busy that we become stiff, stagnant and stressed. We watch television as a form of mindless relaxation. We have to snap out of that and reach past that if you will. That is not living!

Celebrate being alive in this miraculous body! Dance. Move. Sing. Run. Hoop. Jump. Skate. Breathe. Stretch. Even if we are well past the time of being a world class sprinter, **we can all still have a daily time to sit up straight and breathe as deeply as we can a series of times – expanding the lungs and chest.**

Making time to have our own quiet mediation and get some mental exercise. Breathe in new ideas and energy.

A few minutes of deep breathing can help relieve some daily stress and recharge our batteries (for free) with that fresh oxygen in the comfort of our homes. It's better yet if you can go outside among the trees and breathe! Take in some fresh clean air and blow out those old and stagnant toxins deep in the chest. That is a detoxifying exercise that could easily be added to your daily routine. Everyone could take 5 good minutes a day to do that and slowly increase that. Something as simple as breathing is really more gratifying than you think. They even have some cool breathing/meditation apps for smart phones.

Speaking of something everyone can do, try joining a local yoga, Pilates or martial arts class! I highly encourage everyone to check the local Groupons or ask around for recommendations and try something out. Add a new hobby that has beneficial health effects while meeting some new people. Don't think you have to walk in the door super flexible or in shape – there are always a variety of classes accommodating all levels of experience.

Yoga provides a shaping exercise for our internal organs that is pretty unique to yoga poses. It combines the mind and body more than many other forms of physical exercise. It helps to establish and encourage a deep and important connection between our minds and bodies. In fact my beautiful yogi cousin Joy taught me that the word yoga itself means to yoke the mind and body together to work as one.

Martial Arts and its concentrated movements combine mental and physical aspects of exercise all at once as well. That is great for young people to learn to focus and harness the power within – it is a like a moving meditation. It can teach everyone in the family some self-defense techniques – which can be very important – along with some valuable life principles as well. Wax on. Wax off.

We cannot be afraid to try new things. **Maintaining flexibility in our bodies may help us to be more flexible in our minds and mentalities. It can lead to us having a more varied and well-rounded experience in life.**

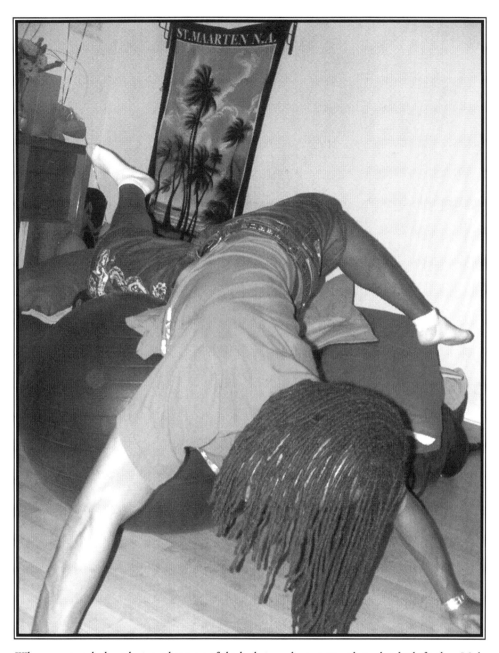

When you stretch, breathe into that part of the body in order to patiently push a little farther. Make it a meditation. Stretch daily.

THE PLANETS & MERCURY RETROGRADE

Astrology is a real science. It is not restricted to the horoscope in the back of the weekly magazines. There is a fascinating world and an undeniable connection we all share with the planets and stars. That connection can be studied and defined through astrology. As they say: as above, so below.

It is hard to get a good perspective in the city nights, but whenever we go out camping or get to escape into nature it is utterly breathtaking how many bright stars literally fill a clear night sky. I can only imagine without all the light pollution and human technology that we have today, how much we would all be captivated by the show of the stars. Astrological science is something we can tune into to receive some real high definition.

I have heard astrology described as the blueprint to the universe. In essence, there is a rotating, tangible form of a 'Bible' above us. That's the place where all those stories originate in the first place. **I would think that an entity as awesome as the Creator would make an everlasting font out of the stars, planets and universe** to relay messages to us. She would do it much bigger than a book. Right?

We need to understand going forward that the planets and their cycles of movement have a substantial effect on us. Gaining some understanding of that is valuable knowledge. It is a very tangible science. It is not "anti-religious" in any way (people sometimes think like that). How can it be? It is *only nature*.

Gazing into the countless night stars and learning about the meanings of their intricate movement and cycles should only further indicate to us the magnificence of our Creator. A better understanding of our outer universe can help us understand our inner universe.

Our ancestors knew exactly how to read that night sky just as plainly as we read articles online. Before there were map apps, the North Star is what provided direction. We have kind of lost touch with that today. I would think we should at least be open to some better understanding of our universe. Hell, we should all be studying it together. It makes sense to utilize all the resources around us. Especially such magnificent (common) resources as the planets and the galaxy!

They only keeps us away from that type of science because it helps to keep us dumbed down and limited. If astrological science is just malarkey, then why do they use it so much and how has it survived all of this time?

The zodiac wheel is literally all over the nations capital. There are 23 zodiacs in public government buildings in Washington, D.C. and many more on the monuments and inside rooms. The National Academy of Science building has a large statue of Albert Einstein overlooking the actual zodiac chart from the date of the statue's dedication (April 22, 1979); it also has the twelve zodiacal characters bronzed on the south entrance door. But yet they never taught us all about astrology in our science classes...*why not?* It is obviously an important part of science.

Even the date that Christians celebrate Easter varies from year to year because it is always the first Sunday after the first full moon that occurs after the **Spring Equinox.** When I was growing up the church's view was that astrology was somehow bad, but that fact about Easter shows me that the religion is to a large degree astrologically based! WTH?

The Bible's parables reference astrology clearly like the Golden Bull story representing Taurus, the Ram representing the new age of Aries and the two fish symbolizing Pisces. Jesus, who is God's son travelling with the 12 Disciples represents the **sun** travelling through the 12 signs and houses of the zodiac. Many religions throughout history all share the same stories, because they have a common source...the stars and the sky above.

All of that shows that astrology is very legitimate and it's something that we should definitely seek to know more about. It is literally a form of higher learning. It is an age-old, mathematical based science that we should be embracing and learning to use as a tool. Many say that the answers to literally everything in life can be found in the Zodiac wheel.

Let's introduce the planets of our solar system and give a quick example of how they can directly affect our daily lives.

DIGABLE PLANETS!

Planet	Gender	Color	Planet of...	Ruler of sign	Mantra
Sun	Masculine	Gold/Orange	Ego/Motive	Leo	"I Will"
Moon	Feminine	White/Silver	Mood/Emotion	Cancer	"I Feel"
Mercury	Masculine	Yellow	Communication/Critical Thinking	Gemini/Virgo	"I Think" & "I Analyze"
Venus	Feminine	Vivid Green/Pink	Morals & Commitments	Taurus/Libra	"I Have" & "I Balance"
Mars	Masculine	Red	Action/Execution	Aries	"I Am"
Jupiter	Feminine	Purple/Violet	Luck/Fortune	Sagittarius	"I See"
Saturn	Feminine	Black/Dark Brown	Discipline/Structure	Capricorn	"I Use"
Uranus	Masculine	Electric Blue	Enlightenment	Aquarius	"I Know"
Neptune	Feminine	Sea Green	Spirituality	Pisces	"I Believe"
Pluto	Feminine	Maroon/Deep Red	Transformation	Scorpio	"I Desire"

The most popular and commonly known example of how the planets above affect us on here on earth is probably the full moon. It's well known that among other things the full moon has a tangible effect on people's behavior. As we see above, the moon controls emotions and mood. We should understand how some of the other planets affect us during their cycles as well.

We can use that knowledge for simple and natural guidelines to help us in our lives. For instance, we should know not to schedule an elective surgery during the full moon time because that is when our blood level is at it's highest. That is just a basic example of how we can apply that higher understanding into our daily lives.

Mercury, the male energy planet that controls communication, periodically provides us with another big example. Three, sometimes four times during the calendar year Mercury goes into a retrograde cycle. That is when it changes its normal pattern and from earth, appears to be spinning backwards. The retrograde periods vary in length, usually lasting at least a few weeks.

The big significance for us is that during the Mercury retrograde period, communication tends to be haywire.

During that time is a big increase of general miscommunication. Items get lost in the mail, calls drop, voice mails get missed and things like that. It's definitely a bad time to make a decision on a big purchase, like buying a home or car. It is also not a good time to sign contracts or begin new ventures. It might not turn out to be the great deal it seemed to be at the time. You want to be sure to **double-check the details** of your travel plans and things like that during the Mercury retrograde period.

Although it sometimes dreaded, this should not be looked at as a negative thing at all – it is just a season. The Retrograde period does have a purpose; it allots a time that we can evaluate things and redirect our energy inside. We should utilize the time for that purpose. My astrology guidebook says it is a great time to do things that begin with the prefix 're' such as: redecorate, reassess, rewrite, restructure and things like that. Mercury retrograde is the time to go back and reflect. The other planets do have retrograde periods as well.

Mercury's retrograde is like a bright yellow sign indicating a sharp curve. It's telling us to shift our focus and readjust things. If we ignore the universal signs and go against the natural grain, it could ultimately just pile on unnecessary stress. Society can sometimes force us to live at a fast pace and ignore the universal speed limit. It is up to us to find ways to stay on nature's course.

It's important for us to know that we have natural tools like this at our disposal. It seems foolish to not take advantage of those FREE and natural guides. Learning how to live in accordance with the universe and nature can ultimately be a vehicle for mastering one's self.

Let's ride.

> "Millionaire's don't use Astrology, *billionaire's* do."
> —J. P. Morgan

You feel me?

CUSTOMIZED BIRTH CHART

Temet Nosce is a Latin phrase that translates to *"Know Thyself"*. Our personal birth charts give us a chance to learn more about our own character traits. Most of us are familiar with only our sun sign, the most commonly referred to sign. But it can be quite interesting and beneficial to have our complete birth chart done. That will identify our moon and rising signs, as well as explain in detail exactly where all of the planets where at our time of birth and how that affects us.

It's very enlightening.

It literally only takes a minute to go online and have our basic birth chart done. Enter the day, exact time and location that you were born and it will quickly give us our own customized birth chart. But the amount of personal insight that you can gain from a session with a skilled astrologist can be nothing short of life changing! I understand that everyone is not into that aspect of life. I'm not asking anyone to live completely by it – but if nothing else, it will surely provide some very interesting insight for us to consider. It is tangible, mathematical science.

What it did for me is give me a clearer idea of how to accept, understand and deal with my own self. I was able to re-affirm my life path and more. It helped me find ways to highlight the strengths in my character and reminds me to address my weaknesses in all aspects of life.

It helps us understand why we approach different parts of our lives in certain ways. Ultimately having our birth charts read will help us learn to understand and master our self – which is something we all need to do. Everyone should have it done at least once. **Get to know your moon and rising signs as well as your sun sign** because they have a big impact on your character as well. Why not utilize those natural tools to learn more about yourself?

*When you are ready to get your chart read, I highly recommend the work of skilled astrologer Krysten Littles. She does an awesome job of patiently reading and enlightening you to the intricacies of your personal zodiac wheel. Check out her website: **thecosmoreport.com** for more information.*

AN INTRODUCTION TO NUMEROLOGY

Before I ran into this menacing thing called Calculus I was planning on majoring in mathematics in college. I had no clue what I wanted to with my life at that time, but I knew that math was universal. Numbers are literally a part of everything in the universe. Every minute and second of each day can be categorized by a specific sequence of numbers.

Numerology is an ancient esoteric science that is based on the symbolism of numbers. The basic idea is that there are only 9 numbers in the universe; each number has a unique vibration that gives it certain properties. Every other number is merely a combination of those 9 numerals. Any sequence of numbers (or letters) can be added and deduced to a single digit; that digit represents the numerological value.

Analyzing our birthday and the other numbers in our numerology chart can help us determine how we fit into the grand equation of this universe. Each person has a unique numerical blueprint. I mention finding our true life's path and purpose a lot in this book; numerology is a tool that will help someone determine their life's purpose.

Much like astrology, numerology is considered a pseudo-science in the Western world. In other parts of the world it is taken much more seriously. It's a basic part of the culture in many places. Certainly these ancient practices have been around this long for a good reason. We have to stop looking at these types of things as weird and realize how valuable they can be.

> *"Men lie. Women lie. Numbers don't."*
>
> —Jay Z

CALCULATE YOUR LIFE PATH NUMBER

Numerologists agree that our **Life Path Number** is the most important number to know and understand. That number is calculated by adding all of the digits of your birthdate down to a single digit. The life path number describes the nature of this journey through life.

First let's examine a few of the characteristics of each number and then we'll do an example calculation.

LPN#	Some Characteristics
1	*The Natural Leader. Independent. Take charge. Good delegator.*
2	*The Nurturer. Diplomatic. Cooperative. Ultimate teammate.*
3	*The Communicator. Creative. Social. Optimistic. Entertainers.*
4	*Builders. Practical. Like structure. Organizer/Planner. Logical.*
5	*The Rebel. Travel. Innovation. Freedom seeker. Change. Progressive thinker.*
6	*Domestic. Family. Duty. Nurturing. Fair. Responsible. Loves home and balance.*
7	*Spiritual. Deep thinker. Isolated types. Loner. Intuitive. Perfectionist. Visionary.*
8	*Hard workers. Very goal orientated, driven. Ambitious. Self-motivated. Wealthy.*
9	*Completion. Wise. Compassionate. Patient. The teacher. Coach. Level mind.*

There isn't room to put a more complete description of the numbers. There are lots of great articles and books out there, plus some great videos on YouTube. After you determine your numbers make sure to investigate it and learn more about it.

The life path number is reached by adding all the numbers of your birthdate down to a single digit. I will take my own birthdate for example:

$$2/19/1973$$
$$2+1+9+1+9+7+3=32$$
$$3+2=\boxed{5}$$

I have a life path number of **5**. Five is the number of change, innovation and freedom. Use this formula to find out the life path number of everyone in your family.

There is only one exception in the calculations and that is the master numbers: 11, 22, 33 and 44. These are special numbers that are not reduced to one digit – they are left whole as 11, 22, 33 or 44. For instance, a person with the birthday 7/11/2000 would just add: 7+11+2. In this case the master number (11) is not broken down (1+1), it remains a whole number (11). This applies to all the master numbers.

Master numbers are very spiritual and represent the extreme of their sum. For instance, 11 would be the very extreme version of the # 2 (1+1=2). The #4 is known as the builders and deals with home or structures; the 22's are known as the master builders, the extreme of 4.

I was not surprised to learn my Life Path Number is 5, which is the roamer. I've always felt a need to see and experience more of the world. This information really helped me come to understand why that is. It helped me embrace my path and focus on finding ways to be productive within it. Relationships or careers that involve lots of travel are ideal situations for person with a life path of 5. Having a more thorough understanding of who you are ultimately helps you relate to others.

Other numbers you might want to know in numerology:

- **Personality Number** – Gives some insight on the "external" you.
- **Destiny Number** – The things you must accomplish to be fulfilled.
- **Heart's Desire/Soul number** – Your inner most desires and dreams.
- **Maturity number** - Indicates the person you will ultimately grow into.

You can get your entire numerology chart done online. It provides more detailed information including the different patterns of life (the 4 Pinnacles, the 4 challenges & the 3 cycles), that are in your chart and breaks things down even further. A skilled numerologist can give you a thorough lesson in what it all means. This information is very enlightening. There is even a **Karmic Debt number** that deals with the debt you come into this life with. The rabbit hole gets pretty deep.

Although this chapter provides only an introduction to numerology, you will find some ways to apply it right away.

SHORTY WHAT YOUR NAME IS?

Your name is much more than just a label. A person sees, hears and writes their name countless times throughout life. We grow to truly embody our names. Our birth name is used to calculate some of the other numbers in our numerology chart.

The letters of the alphabet have a corresponding number value. To calculate your Destiny number, add the value of your full birth name down to one digit. The destiny number in numerology is all about your natural talents, skills, strengths and weaknesses at birth.

The Numerical Value of Letters

1	2	3	4	5	6	7	8	9
A	B	C	D	E	F	G	H	I
J	K	L	M	N	O	P	Q	R
S	T	U	V	W	X	Y	Z	

Remember we want to add the entire birth name down to a single digit, for my name it would look like this:

Raymond	Jonathan	Stone
9 1 7 4 6 5 4	1 6 5 1 2 8 1 5	1 2 5 5 5

9+1+7+4+6+5+4= 36	1+6+5+1+2+8+1+5= 28	1+2+5+5+5= 18
3+6=9	2+8 = 10	1+8= 9
	1+0 = 1	

9	**1**	**9**

9+1+9=19

1+9 =10

1+0= **1**

After adding all the letters in my name down to one digit I arrive at my Destiny number of 1. Calculate your destiny number and see what you may be able to learn from it. Remember that everyone is born to be great at something. Share your gifts with us all.

The **Personality number** is calculated by adding the values of only the **consonants** in your name. That number represents the parts of yourself that you are most ready and willing to reveal.

The **Soul** (or Heart's Desire) **number** is calculated by adding the values of _only_ the **vowels** in your name down to one digit. That number represents your true desires. It is said to be the reason behind the choices you make in all areas of life. The soft sounds of the vowels represent your more inner, subconscious desires.

The **Birthday number** is found by adding the day of your birth down to one digit. Mine for example, the 19th would be: 1+9=10 drop the 0 and my birthday number then is **1**.

It is true that someone can change their name. Changing your name would be creating a different vibration and number value. Keep in mind that it may not be an overnight thing. It will likely take a while to embody the new vibration. From now on if you are going to change your name, it makes sense to know the numerology of the new name. This gives you something else to consider when you're naming your children too!

It makes sense to check the numbers on any variation of your name or different nicknames. After doing my full name I also did the name that most people know me as, which is **Ray Stone**. I find myself doing the numbers on everything: addresses, phone numbers, parking space numbers and any sequence of numbers since I've been exposed to numerology.

Use the system to stay in synch with the flow of the universe. Pay attention to the numbers of the month, for example January 2015: 1+2+0+1+5 = **9**. 9 represents completion; maybe that is the time to schedule the completion of a big project that you are working on. We also know that the following month February 2015 will be a **1**. 1 is a good time for new beginnings. Following the numbers can provide an organized way to forecast, anticipate and plan for things.

It might be best to meditate during the 7 o'clock hour of the day; the number 7 vibrates spirituality. This is an example of a practical way numerology can be applied to your day-to-day life.

The best day to plan a small home improvement project is a '4' day because the number 4 deals with structure and the home. Once you open yourself to it, this stuff starts to make a lot of sense!

I think the true enlightenment for us in modern times is learning how to incorporate the ancient practices into our everyday existence. We have been disconnected from these things for too long. Our ancestors knew how to incorporate and apply all of these ideals. It served as a guide throughout their lives. I recently learned that the best time to shop for home décor is when the Moon (or Venus) is in the sign of Cancer. Cancer is the 4th sign of the zodiac; we know that the #4 deals with the home. The symmetry of it all makes it easy to grasp.

The best time to shop for groceries is when the Moon is in Cancer or Virgo, which deals with health and attention to details. A good time to shop for clothes is when the moon is in Leo, the sign that rules clothing. These are free and simple guides that we have right at our disposal, yet we generally don't utilize them. The universe has set these patterns for us. Simply learning how to follow them might be the key to mastering life in the Matrix. Numerology can play a huge part in the understanding and mastery of life.

Have you ever noticed how sometimes you keep seeing the same combination of numbers over and over again? That happens to everybody right? When the same numbers keep catching your eye, it is not just a coincidence. No! That is actually the universe attempting to communicate with you. It's trying to send you signs and messages through those numbers. Wow! Isn't that just amazing? Learning about numerology can show you brand new ways to approach life. That is a class to sign up for!

And to think…I was wasting all that time stressing over a damn Calc class. Ha!

THE POWER OF WORDS

All of my books end with a bonus section dealing with vocabulary. I love words!

ELYGAD ended with love vs. h*te. It reminded us how speaking and focusing on what we like and love allows us to attract positive experiences. When we do that, the universe gives us more things to love. If we constantly complain about we do not care for, we will only see more and more of that. **We speak things into existence.**

We discussed how we should use more of our vocabulary. There are many other words that we can use to describe the way we feel about things. Today we are in the habit of saying h*te for the most trivial things. That too is a result of us being products of our environment. Naturally we say the words and phrases that we hear around us all the time.

This section talks more about the power of our words and how they can affect us. It also will show us a **more complete way to utilize the dictionary.**

Dr. Masaru Emotu is a famous Japanese author/scientist who did some amazing studies centered on words and water. Take a little time to get familiar with his studies. He illustrated with photographs exactly how words and intention can change the actual structure of water molecules.

For instance, in one experiment he put the word "HATE" on a piece of paper, placed it in a jar and put it in a body of water, froze it, and took pictures of the shape of the molecules. The word hate in the water made it an ugly and confused picture.

While the word "LOVE" in the same water produced a beautiful crystal shaped molecule structure. That points out how the water somehow knew and reacted instantly and directly to the energy of the words. Amazing! Dr. Emotu continued his research for many years and has published several books. It is very interesting reading, be sure to check them out.

So how does that even happen? Water can't read, can it? Somehow the water can feel the vibration and intention of the words.

My vaporizer reminded me in a private conversation one night that we already know very well that our words carry a strong vibration with them.

We say it ourselves. You know how we talk in the hood, it's not enough to ask somebody do they hear you, no – you ask, "do you feel me?" Without any physical contact, we are asking if can you feel our words! Or we might say a very foul mouth person is 'cussing up a storm' – even that is some indication how words indeed effect the climate and environment in the room.

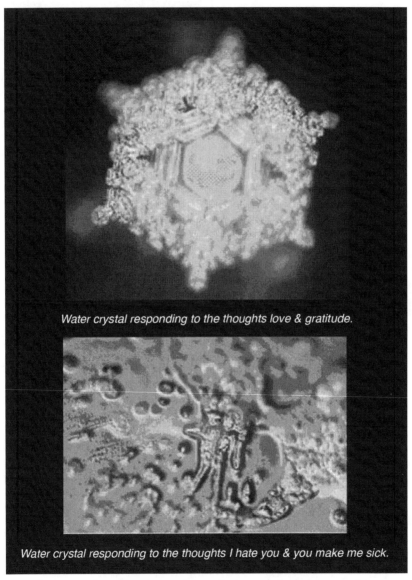

Water crystal responding to the thoughts love & gratitude.

Water crystal responding to the thoughts I hate you & you make me sick.

That is a clear visual indication of just how much power and impact there actually is in our words. Our bodies are vessels composed mainly of water, so it is safe to assume that our internal water is constantly reacting to different words, energies and vibrations. We just may not realize it is happening.

Products of Our Environment

Looking at that picture and understanding that our bodies are 78% water – one has to wonder the effect on us internally when we are saying the word "h*te" repetitively? Our blood is 92% water. Our brains are 75% water. Things like that **could be having a profound impact on our physical health and state of mind.** Gaining control of the energy that comes out of our being is a good thing, because what we put out is what returns back to us. That is universal law.

Watching so much violence on tell-lie-vision and the harsh world of the music industry could be really upsetting our internal organs. Those loud talking people that are always complaining and negatively gossiping about people – who we say *'make us sick'* – could literally be helping to make us sick, you know? It is a good idea to stay around pleasant people who vibrate harmonic energy through our internal waters.

The Dictionary & Etymology
When we look up a word in the dictionary we usually look at the meanings of it and that's it. Maybe we read the sample sentences too. One part that we overlook is the origin and original meaning of word – the **etymology**. It can be very interesting and eye opening to learn the original meaning of some words that we use frequently in conversation.

Here is an example:
A word like "**nice**" – is something that we say and hear all the time. Around children we will say things like, "Now you all play **nice**," or "don't you hit him! Be *nice*".

It is also used in other ways like, 'that's a **nice** whip bro'. On the east coast they might say 'yo, this kid is **nice**' on the court or microphone'.

So we look it up in the dictionary and we basically know already how nice is defined. It reads as follows:

Nice
-adjective, *nic-er, nic-est.*
    1. pleasing; agreeable; delightful: a nice visit
    2. amiably pleasant; kind: they are always nice to strangers.

Of course we get pretty familiar with and learn those meanings. The part that is not on the vocabulary quizzes, and that we tend to overlook is the etymological information. It is not even included in every dictionary anymore. It is the information that is in bold inside of [**brackets**] ~ which I used to totally ignore.

This is how the word 'nice' is defined within the brackets:

[**Origin:** 1250-1300; ME (middle English): **foolish, stupid** < OF: **silly, simple** < L nescius **ignorant, incapable**]

One very old, thick dictionary I ran across also had included these now obsolete meanings with the others:

13. Obsolete. **Coy, shy, reluctant**
14. Obsolete. **Unimportant; trivial.**

Wow. See how interesting that is? These are definitely not things that we want our children to be or to play like!

But that is the origin of the word and the original meaning and was the initial energy behind it. Of course we do not say it with that in mind. We mean something totally different when we say it. But since that is clearly the original energy of the word – one has to wonder if that remains a part of it to some degree. It was created with that intention.

It is something that we have to consider. I'd love to have a discussion with Dr. Emotu about that (when I get some people, I'm gonna have my people get with his people).

After learning about this, I can definitely see some very well to do type of people looking down their nose at some servant and saying, "oh you shouldn't have – that is so **nice** of you."

While it sounds good, they really mean it in the sense of silly and simple. Foolish. I'm thinking that could be part of the reason they say '*nice*' guys finish last too – right?

I laugh at myself because now instinctively, almost every time someone says 'nice' around me, I mumble ever so softly to myself, *"nice means stupid."*

Another interesting word, that is even arguably more popular than nice is "bad". We say and hear 'bad' all the time. Kids and bad just go together.

If a child is throwing food on the floor, being really stubborn and not behaving we are quick to say, "oooh he or she is being **bad!**"

I see parents hold their babies, smiling and totally innocently asking "why are you so bad huh?"

> **Bad**
> (slang) bad-der, bad-dest
> -adjective
> 1. not good in any manner or degree.
> 2. Having wicked or evil character; morally reprehensible: There is no such thing as a bad boy.
> 3. Of poor or inferior quality; defective; deficient: a bad diamond. A bad spark plug.

Right. But once again, we go inside the brackets.

> [**Origin**: 1250-1300; ME (middle English bade, perh. OE (old English) **hermaphrodite, or womanish man**]

!!!

It is right there in your dictionary. Go look. That is crazy right? I never paid ANY attention to that part before.

When I was first taught this I remember thinking about Michael Jackson. He sang over and over again, "I'm bad, I'm bad – I'm really, really bad".

Don't get me wrong, I love me some Michael Jackson – rest in peace to the greatest entertainer that ever did it! Hands down. But we all saw that he did become really **bad**, in the original sense of the word – a womanish man.

In today's time there are more gay men in our community than ever before. Even the so-called thugs (bad boys) of today walk around with their asses hanging completely out like that is somehow hard! Am I suggesting that the excessive usage of the word is the reason behind that? No, not necessarily. Although I do think it might be something worth taking into consideration.

What we do know for sure is that we can speak things into existence and there is great power in our words. This information made me much more conscientious of the words and phrases that I use regularly. I also listen more carefully these days.

I've caught myself actually saying things like "...man my head is killing me!" But I had to get rid of that habit. That is not what I mean. What I mean is more like my head is uncomfortable, but it is not killing me. I don't want it to either. I've become a whole lot more aware of the words and phrases that I use. It is easy to fall into saying what we hear everyone around us saying. We should scrutinize the things that come out of our mouths. As Dr. Emoto's work confirms, words are powerful.

Having some understanding the origin of words will help us develop a better understanding of language in general. All law is based on contracts. Understanding the elements of a contract is vitally important. Knowing how to read and write the language of the system is the (red pill) key to finding freedom within it. In business and in every aspect of life, effective communication is very paramount. Vocabulary is very important.

The combinations of words we use is actually us casting spells...what spells are you casting daily? Practice using phrases with a purpose, for instance: resist saying you are not going to "try" to do something – instead know that you are going to do it. Don't start off sentences with the words "I can't..." – it already limits you right out of the gate. Focus on stating the things you can and will do.

When you read the Constitution of the United States or a law dictionary you will see just how important knowing the actual meaning of words is. This whole matrix system is built on the clever manipulation of terminology. For instance in legal terms, a **_motor vehicle_** and an **_automobile_** are two completely different things. Which one do you drive? And exactly which one are you: a **_driver_**, an **_operator_** or a **_traveler_**? Although they sound similar, they have very different legal meanings. That list goes on and on. It is a very good idea to get familiar with simple civics and understand the law of the land. The school systems conveniently skip over all of that. And as they always remind us, ignorance of the law is no excuse.

One last note on etymology and example of just how in tuned the ancients were with the stars is this: the word **consider** etymologically means to examine the stars. So before making a decision about something like planning an event, one would first consider the placement of the stars and planets. Just like you should reconsider signing a contract during Mercury's retrograde. The etymology of the word **disaster** is: to not consult the stars – the translation is an *'ill-starred'* event. Meaning that the event was planned without considering the stars. That is was a disaster by definition. That is how important astrology was at that time in history.

I thought that all of this was something definitely worth sharing, knowing that it will provoke some thought in my beloved readers. That's the reason I started Ra One Pubs! I encourage you to investigate and look into some of these things for yourself. Question everything. There is a whole lot to be learned outside of the proverbial box.

I look forward to returning with more info next time. I hope that your waters were making a most beautiful picture as you read this book. It was prepared for you with the utmost peace and love. Namaste.

<u>Highly Recommended Reading</u>

Cleaning Yourself to Death: How Safe is Your Home? by Pat Thomas

What's in This Stuff? by Pat Thomas

Twinkie, Deconstructed by Steve Ettlinger

Worms Eat My Garbage by Mary Appelhof

Arm & Hammer Baking Soda: Over 100 Helpful Household Hints by Christine Halvorson

Heinz Vinegar: Over 100 Helpful Household Hints by Christine Halvorson

100,000,000 Guinea Pigs: Dangers in Everyday Foods, Drugs, and Cosmetics by Arthur Kallet and F.J. Schlink

Toxic Beauty: How hidden chemicals in cosmetics harm you by Dawn Mellowship

Urban Kryptonite & The Ancient 20 by Damien McSwine

SKIN DEEP: The essential guide to what's really in the toiletries and cosmetics you use by Pat Thomas

The Flouride Deception by Christopher Bryson

Nutritional Healing: A Practical A to Z Reference to Drug-Free Rememdies Using Vitamins, Minerals, Herbs & Food Supplements by Phyllis A. Balch

Llewellyn's (Annual) Daily Planetary Guide by Llewellyn

The Feng Shui Bible by Simon Brown

Crystal Prescriptions: The A – Z guide to over 1,200 symptoms and their healing crystals by Judy Hall

The Toxic Bomb: Can the Mercury in Your Dental Fillings Poison You? by Sam Ziff

Juice Fasting & Detoxification: Use the Healing Power of Fresh Juice to Feel Young and Look Great The fastest way to restore your health by Steve Meyerowitz

Official Slavery by Dr. Brian Lucas

Redemption in Law (Theory and Practice): Cracking the Code, 2nd Edition by BBCOA

The Constitution of the United States & The Constitution of Your State

Black's Law Dictionary

A FEW MORE GOOD BRANDS!

I hope that this book prompts readers to look beyond the commercial retailers for local products and other options. Remember that there are natural versions of all the commercial products that we use. Here is a list of brands that go the extra step to make their products the natural way – perfect alternatives to the chemically laced norm. Upgrades. Remember to seek and support the local producers in your area.

Kiss My Face soap	Shampoo, deodorant, moisturizer
Dudu Osun	Raw African Black Soap
Diva Cup	Menstrual Cups
Nubian Heritage	Soap, lotion
Emerita	Female hygiene products, lubricants
Entwine Couture	Natural hair care and styling
African Republic	Shea butter, shea nut oil
Berjohs Natural Hair & Skin	All Natural Hair & Skin care products
Mi Mi's Natural	Natural Products That Care about you!
Auromere	Toothpaste, mouthwash, facial mud, shampoo/conditioner
Vadik	Ayurvedic products: neti pot, nasal oil
Earth's Beauty	Lipstick, mascara, eye shadow/pencils, blush
Suncoat Cosmetics	Liquid foundation, hair styling gel, mascara
Natra Care	Non-chlorinated menstrual pads, maternity products
Aura Cassia	Essential oils, cocoa butter
Out Of Africa	Shea Butter, lip balm lotion, body wash, body oil
Star Essence	Spritzer, sprays
Dherbs	Herbal cleanses, extracts, elixirs, inspirants
Himalayan Institute	Neti pot, neti-stick, sinus spray
Zenzele	A natural hair and body movement
Eco-Dent	Chewing gum
Sundial	African man-back, woodroot tonic, ashanti weight loss
Nature's Baby Organic	Baby powder, lotion, shampoo
Songhai	Liquid black soap
Organic Grooming	Soap, men's shaving cream, deodorant
Trace minerals	Liquid ionic vitamins and minerals (for adults & children)
Auromere	Toothpaste, mouthwash, conditioner, shampoo
Primal Pit Paste	All natural deodorant options for adults and youth!
Holistic Heights	Natural and electrical health, beauty & wellness products.

I really want to thank all the local producers of natural products. Thank you for filling an important void in our communities. Please support local producers and artist. Pay a little more if you have to, understanding the safety and value of knowing the source. Say goodbye to all the beauty supply, drug store products filled with the common poisons!

Products of Our Environment

For those who might not know:

GLOSSARY TERMS

Spring Equinox – The Equinox refers to the two days of the year when the sun passes the celestial equator. On the day of the Spring Equinox there is exactly 12 hours of daylight and 12 hours of darkness. This occurs right around the 20th of March.

Summer Solstice – After the spring Equinox, the daylight is slowly increased and it is light outside longer than it is dark. That continues throughout the summer then finally until the Summer Solstice, which marks the longest day of the year. It occurs in June between the 20th and 22nd. After that the days will gradually get shorter.

Autumn Equinox – The same as the Spring Equinox above, on this day there is an equal amount of daylight and night hours. 12/12. It occurs right around October 22nd.

Winter Solstice - After the Autumn Equinox, the days gradually get shorter and shorter. It is dark longer than it is light outside. That continues until the Winter Solstice, which is the longest night of the year. That is a day with the least amount of daylight hours. It is in December around the 21st.

Chakras   – Energy centers inside the body in which energy flows through.

There are 7 Chakras:

> **The Root Chakra** @ the base of the spine
> **The Sacral Chakra** @ the lower abdomen
> **The Solar Plexus Chakra** @ the upper abdomen
> **The Heart Chakra** @ Center of chest just above the heart
> **The Throat Chakra** @ the throat
> **The Third Eye Chakra** @ The forehead between the eyes
> **The Crown Chakra** @ the very top of the head

PLANT GOOD SEEDS

Grow some food of our own this season. Here are some sources of good heirloom seeds. These could prove to be very valuable resources in the near future as the corporations are attempting to flood and control the world with their Genetically Modified industrial seeds. The American Government and federal agencies are on the wrong team.

This is the time to return to the old fashioned way of growing our own food and sharing/trading with friends, family and neighbors. Up to date information and a more complete local listings can be found online, here are a few good heirloom seed sources that are GMO-free. (courtesy of www.ruralspin.com) Support your local farmers and those doing things the right way:

Baker Greek Heirloom Seeds:	www.rareseeds.com
Bountiful Gardens:	www.bountifulfardens.org
Heirloom Seeds:	www.heirloomseeds.com
Heirloom Tomatoes:	www.heriloomtomatoes.net
Heritage Harvest Seed:	www.heritageharvestseed.com
Johnny's Selected Seeds:	www.johnnyseeds.com
Kusa Seed Society:	www.ancientcerealgrains.com
Landreth Seed company:	www.landrethseeds.com
Living Seed Complany:	www.livingseedcompany.com
Native Seeds:	www.nativeseeds.org
Seed Savers Exchange:	www.seedsavers.org
Solana Seeds:	www.solanaseeds.netfirms.com
Southern Exposure Seed Exchange:	www.southernexposure.com
Sustainable Seed Company:	www.sustainableseedco.com
Territorial Seed:	www.territorialseed.com
Victory Seed Company:	www.victoryseeds.com

Remember to look for local CSA's (Community Supported Agriculture) and Buying Clubs – two of the newer ways to conveniently get real, old-fashioned fruits and veggies to your family.

FACEBOOK PAGES/WEBSITES:

* Learning New Skills for Survival

* Herbs and Oils World

* Holistic Heights

* VeganHoodTV

* Supanova Slom

* Love Earth Herbal

* Chef Ahki

* The Cosmo Report

* Preserving Community

* Millions Against Monsanto

* RBG Fit Club * Restored Inc. (Detoxification of the Mind, Body & Spirit.)

* Changing the Definitionof Murder to include Animals   * The Healing Spoon

* Trying to Eat, Drink and Bathe in something that wont kill me * The Moon Ministry

* Food MythBusters (The real story about what we eat)   * Act Naturally

* Center for Science in the the Public interest   * Opare Integrative Health

* http://sosjuice.com/foodfight

* Veggie Love Planet

Contact Ra One Publications:

Ray Stone is available for **demonstrations, lectures, life-coaching packages, awesome kitchen makeovers and private consultations.**

The consultations are awesome and can help you jumpstart a complete transition in your family with just a few customized and easy steps. Move forward on a new, healthier path. We would love to help you!

Website:	www.ra1pubs.com
Twitter:	@Ra1pubs
Instagram:	ra1pubs
Email:	ra1publications@gmail.com
Phone:	313.559-6200

WORDS FROM THE AUTHOR

I am the classic Piscean dreamer. It is quite typical for the Pisces to often swim away, off into our own little dream worlds. The lower side of the sign can get stuck there. Only existing in that world like the movie Inception, drinking like a 'fish', wishing it was actually reality. We can even pity ourselves and get depressed that everyone cannot see things the clear way that we do. But the higher side of the sign is actually able to emerge from that dream world, with something tangible to offer everyone that will actually help create it. At times, I have surely been both of those fish. Through my work in life and Ra One Publications I hope to achieve the latter.

This is my second offering towards creating a new world – my second dream coming true. As I was pulling this book together, I realized that most of the material dates way back to 2008! I became quite frustrated with myself realizing how long it has taken me to get this information out here. But, in my trademark optimism, I figure hey…better late than never. Besides I know that time is only an illusion. Things always happen in their proper season. I really want to encourage all the light workers out here working towards their dreams to **keep pushing** because this is manifestation season! You can create exactly the reality you want!

I will always give thanks for and cherish my mom **Lois Stone**. All throughout my life she encouraged me to let me let my mind travel. I played dead serious games of one-on-none basketball with a ball of aluminum foil in our tiny living room. When I woke up really early she'd take me on these magical boat rides that served special treats. The boat was right on the floor in the front room while playing classical music. She had me pause all the time appreciate the brilliant blue sky, smell fresh air, listen to the birds communicating and admire beautiful flowers. She wanted me to appreciate the magic of nature. I hear her doing the same thing with my niece and nephews. They don't really know that they appreciate it yet. She was always teaching me to think beyond and dream big. She definitely needed another Pisces child. We are a custom fit.

I was never just in that little duplex, on that block, in that concrete jungle – I was always gone. Imagining, visualizing, reading, wondering, wandering and pondering – that's what my mom had always taught me to do since way back then. Now, after a lifetime of practice, I am manifesting my dreams. I put things out in the universe and watch them unfold right before my eyes. (You are holding and reading one of my visualizations right now). This makes life so exciting – it's like a magic carpet ride. For this ride and truly for everything I learn, accomplish and share with you all in this lifetime, I owe great thanks to my Mom! I appreciate all the time you took to instill so many things in me. Thank you. I love you so much.

I want to send my love and strength to all the moms out here raising our future leaders. It is the most important job in the world. We live in a society where our women are vastly underappreciated. I want to pay my respect to all the Queens of the earth. Thank you all.

ACKNOWLEDGEMENTS

I should first give thanks and pay my respect to all of the many people that I have studied and learned from, including (but not limited to): **Dick Gregory, Dejuty Ma'at Ra, Bob Marley, Dr. Sebi, Kevin Trudeau, Dr. B Sirius, Malcolm X, Alex Jones, Osho, Michael Pollan, Vandana Shiva, Taj Tarek Bey, Sabir Bey, Kenya K. Stevens, Krysten Littles, Hakim Bey, Derrick Stallings, Queen Afua, Bill Maher, Jessica Care Moore, Dr. Emotu, George Carlin, Dr. Jewel Pookrum, Dead Prez, KRS One, Chef Ahki, David Wolfe, Dr. Thomas Lodi, Jonathan Foer, Dr. Laila Afrika, Eric Schlosser, Dr. T. Colin Campbell & Thomas M Campbell II, Dr. Lorraine Keefa and Dr. Isis**. Thank you all for being great examples and resources when I was out there really searching for alternatives and answers.

My entire family has always been a great source of education itself. I see greatness and great intelligence all throughout my family on all levels. Seeing my **brother, uncles, aunts** and **cousins** own and operate their own businesses (and hustles), gave me the confidence to jump out here. It helped to widen my realm of possibilities. I'm very blessed and proud to come from such a talented and charismatic family. It has always given me confidence and a strong sense of security. I never take that for granted. I appreciate all my **Beard** family and extended family! I love you all! We HAVE to get a family tattoo already what's going on!?! Love you Sydney, Chris and Chase ~ all my heart.

CC…I remember one of the many magical holiday seasons that you brought the Matrix to Detroit on DVD – or maybe it was still VHS way back then. I didn't know anything about it. We watched it over and over and it was better every time. We had so many 'screenings' and discussions about it with our families, Bams and everyone else. That movie (and those times) was life changing! It was a Zeitgeist like slap in the face. Since then my mind was open to a brand new level. That was the red pill. When I was writing this book I realized that you were actually the very first to put me up on Mercury retrograde too. Way before I was even into it. That was yet another door down a lifelong hallway…thanks for being my Trinity.

Thanks to brother Dejuty Ma'at Ra, and the entire staff at Dhealthstore for your support. Dejuty thanks for the thorough education you offer through videos and writing. Dhealthstore is a tremendous resource! I want to make it clear that there is not any financial or any other reason that I support his products other than the fact that I totally believe in them. The videos & products are amazing! He is dropping knowledge in ALL areas of life. I will always strongly encourage everyone to support his stuff because I know his products carry that loving, healing energy inside. There is high quality and integrity in both their products and service.

POE and *ELYGAD* both urge us to either **be** the source or *know* the source of the products we use going forward. **Please get to know dhealthstore.com** and you will find it is an awesome resource to help facilitate moving away from using poisonous chemical cosmetics/medicines for good! They have a huge selection of herbal formulas and herbs, even rare exotic ones. Don't dare go to the beauty supply store to get anything before you check this place out. The prices are unbelievably reasonable. They really do serve the people with great sales offers literally all the time, plus senior/student discounts. Please check it out.

Much love to my Ra One Publications production team of **Michael Angelo Chester** (graphic design) and **Ann Houston** (editor) I appreciate your help getting this project presentable for my readers – many thanks to you both. I look forward to working with you both in the future. Let's keep this thing going. I love my team. I want to thank **Dana** from digital and everyone at **McNaughton & Gunn**. M & G has been very supportive and provided excellent customer service over the years – even for a tiny press like ours.

Big thanks to my dear friend **Roxanne Moore** – thank you for always being down to discuss projects and provide that key input under pressure. I always appreciate your encouragement. You hear all about my manifestations and see them they come true. I really appreciate the encouragement. **Diana Felix Ed. D,** your understanding and timely encouragement really helped re-energize me and got me back on my 'change the world' grind a few years back. You still have a permanent seat on your committees. Sorry about your mom.

Ra One Pubs supports the spread of real knowledge. Special shout out to brother **Sabir Bey** and the entire staff over at **LA Talk Live** – thanks for putting me on the **Sabir Bey Show** team and putting that real information out here. They do not provide us with a proper education in schools, and they tell us bullshit in the mainstream media. That show and station are great platforms to present some real important information. Unfiltered. Tune in for some real edutainment and have your notebook ready. Special thanks to the beautiful and ultra talented **Rhona "Rho" Bennet** at LA Talk Live as well, thank you for your support! Peace and love to my brother **Shakim, Grand Master Jerry Bell, Rich** on the boards and my unofficial enlightener **Cosmo Krys.**

Instead of being too personal, let me just say special thanks to <u>everyone</u> out there that supported the *ELYGAD* project. I love and appreciate too many people to list. I sincerely thank you all! All the stores who carry **Ra One** books – thank you so much. It is still a big thrill for me to walk in and see my imagination on the shelf. Knowing that my words and thoughts are out in the universe working is indescribable – I have some great ideas coming soon! Ra One Publications is going to do some great things! All the encouraging feedback

I've gotten is really what keeps me going. Thank you, thank you, and thank you.

I love you so much **Deegie**! Always. You really accept me for who I am and I really appreciate that. I bet you're a 9! Ha. Stay sweet and special **Aziza** (Chef Z) – love you and your fam. Shot to my brother Samir, your crib doubled as my high-rise office many times in the D. Thanks to the roots man **DJ Moses**. Pack it up and move to the islands to play music already bro! Wassup with that **DJ Skeez?**☺ Peace **Woodward Walker. Tasneem. Kemit!... Kouns. Yak!** Hugs little **Nova**. Extra special thanks to my Mia/Oak family **Ethan** and **Kim** I love you both! Thanks for holding me completely down in a tough time! I really appreciate that, it means a lot to me. **DeMetria**...you too. I'm excited to see your powerful book to come out and help so many people. I'm proud of you. Thanks for being a beautiful guardian angel. **Nina**...thanks for the years of friendship, holding me down and showing me some amazing parts of the earth. I appreciate you.

Congrats and all the best wishes to my peeps **Kaaren** and **Moncho**! Same to my dear, dear friend **Kamila**! I love you. Congrats to you and **Mardy**. I'm happy for you all. My family **Cassandra Kimble** and **Sandra Elliot**, thanks for all your support, y'all be sharing those *ELYGAD*'s posts for me! Lol! Thank you so much. My cousin **Rush**, who actually put me up on 3D printing, and **Blanca** thanks for letting me feature precious little **Avery** in that pic. Love you both. Thank you **Harriet**, your place provided me a perfect writing hideaway filled with **Alan**'s brilliant spirit. I appreciate you! **Asya**, thank you for your support it means a lot to me. I really admire the way you follow the stars too!

Ok...I'm tripping. I want to name, thank and bear hug ALL the many people who have helped me ~ I better save some for the next book though. Nobody really reads this far in the book anyway. Lol!

jCm...quoted your butt. Lol. I'll always be a big fan of your revolutionary work. I have seen first hand how tirelessly you work to pull things together. I'm inked on the list of the many that you inspire, thanks for being a friend & my family. Can't wait till your albums drop! **King**...you inspire me more than anyone man. I really can't put words together to explain how much I love you and appreciate being a part of your life. I'm so anxious to see all the things that you have to offer this world. We have some classics in our catalog already.

Brother **Sid** (**Nsa Kabenga Kaisi Maceo Guevara**) your brilliant words couldn't have reached me at a more perfect time. I just so appreciate you taking the time to do that man. On my darkest days, I know I can lean on your review to remind me that it is worth it to keep grinding. I'll always be grateful for that man. You are a really gifted person and writer in my eyes! Peace and love to you. Thanks again.

DEFINITIONS FROM BLACK'S LAW DICTIONARY
(4th Pocket Edition)

---

person.   (13c) 1. A human being.

artificial person. (17c) An entity, such as a corporation, created by law and given certain legal rights and duties of a human being; a being, real or imaginary, who for the purpose of legal reasoning is treated more or less as a human being.

Way back in the day my mom was so happy that her precious youngest child was born. Such a joyous moment it is, the beginning of a person's life. Everybody in the family is happy and congratulatory. My cousins tease that my mom wouldn't let anyone within 10 feet of me as a baby. She said I was too precious.

My sister Pam was happy too! She had helped my mom pick the name. They determine that I will be known as **Raymond Jonathan Stone**. "He's gonna do something very special in his life," my aunt Tish prophesized. She saw something in me. She said she could tell I was a special **person**.

What happens next is the real life Matrix shit. A human being was born – but to add to the commerce game of this country, an artificial person was created that very same day. The law dictionary definitions above clearly show the difference between the two. The precious little **person** – the baby human being (labeled 13c) Raymond Jonathan Stone, subsequently becomes the little artificial corporate (often referred to as **strawman**) entity (labeled 17c), it will be called: **RAYMOND JONATHAN STONE**.

Do you see the difference in those two? I do. The one at the bottom is the one on ALL of my bills, tickets and shit like that. That is the one on State ID's & driver's license, birth certificate, passport, credit card and phone bills – as a matter of fact, it's on the majority of the mail I receive in all-caps that way. WTF? That is not the way my family wrote it.

All the bills are addressed to the all-capital version of me because all the agreements and applications (which are posing as contracts) that I sign…I am really signing not on behalf of myself, the person (Raymond Jonathan Stone).

Legally, I am acting **NOT** as a human being; I am acting as that corporate entity that it clearly states is treated more or less like a human being – the artificial person (17c).

In the beginning of this book I talked about our behavior patterns in regards to us buying & replacing commercial products just the way the corporations want us to. In the end you see, we are not only behaving like the corporations would want us to, we actually ARE acting as corporations. Artificial people. Artificial world. Welcome to the artificial world.

That's a quick peak into a very deep rabbit hole – but it's also a really simple concept. Don't take anything from me, I'm only pointing things out. You have to draw your own conclusions, if any. I just wanted to give a little more food for thought and close out with this – only for those who want to go there. For anyone seeking moor information, I can help point you in the right direction, but the info is definitely out here. Use your smartphone for something smart. This is the information age and so it is readily available if you seek it and you are open to it. Most things we need to know, we already know. What we need to learn is how to block out all the distractions of the world and listen to our inner voice.

Anti-Corporation
(In Propria Persona)

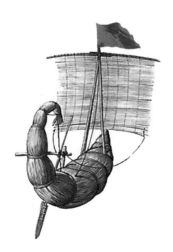